AIDS

A Communication Perspective

COMMUNICATION

A series of volumes edited by
Dolf Zillmann and **Jennings Bryant**

AIDS

A Communication Perspective

Edited by

Timothy Edgar
University of Maryland, College Park

Mary Anne Fitzpatrick
University of Wisconsin, Madison

Vicki S. Freimuth
University of Maryland, College Park

LEA **LAWRENCE ERLBAUM ASSOCIATES, PUBLISHERS**
1992 **Hillsdale, New Jersey**   **Hove and London**

Lawrence Erlbaum Associates, Inc., Publishers
365 Broadway
Hillsdale, New Jersey 07642

Library of Congress Cataloging-in-Publication Data

AIDS : a communication perspective / edited by Timothy Edgar, Mary
   Anne Fitzpatrick, Vicki S. Freimuth.
      p.   cm. — (Communication)
   Includes bibliographical references and index.
   ISBN 0-8058-0998-8
   1. AIDS (Disease)—Prevention.   2. Health risk communication.
3. Health behavior.   I. Edgar, Timothy.   II. Fitzpatrick, Mary
Anne, 1949–   .   III. Freimuth, Vicki S.   IV. Series: Communication
(Hillsdale, N.J.)
   RA644.A25A2863   1992
   614.5'993—dc20   91-44036
                                                              CIP

Printed in the United States of America
10   9   8   7   6   5   4   3   2

*This book is dedicated to our friend and colleague,
Robert W. Norton, for his pioneering work on
communication and AIDS*

Contents

Preface

As the number of AIDS cases multiplied throughout the early and mid-1980s, it became apparent that no cure or vaccine was on the horizon. Prevention through appropriate behavior was, and still is, the best weapon available to fight further spread of HIV infection. However, individuals take necessary actions to prevent a disease such as AIDS only when (a) they are properly informed and (b) they feel motivated to respond to the information they possess. In order to achieve a clearer understanding of these two facets of the prevention process, we must examine the interplay of the messages individuals receive about AIDS at the public level and the messages exchanged between individuals at the interpersonal level.

In November 1987 at the Speech Communication Association conference in Boston, Professors Robert Norton and Jim Hughey organized a small, informal meeting of researchers interested in communication issues related to AIDS. Since that time, a growing number of communication scholars have developed research tracks devoted to AIDS concerns. In order to encourage the exchange of ideas and to disseminate research results, a variety of forums developed. For example, the Health Communication Division of the International Communication Association sponsored an AIDS mini-conference in New Orleans in 1988. Special issues of *AIDS and Public Policy Journal* and *Communication Research* provided outlets for AIDS-related research in 1989 and 1990 respectively. And in November 1991 a team of communication scholars was invited to the

Centers for Disease Control in Atlanta to discuss communication research trends and directions with government health officials.

This book represents an extended link in the information chain. The specific purpose of the book is to examine how theory informs our understanding of communication processes as they relate to the AIDS crisis in the United States and other parts of the world. As we and the other contributors to the book explore the issue from a variety of theoretical and conceptual viewpoints, we hope to stimulate thought that will lead to the pragmatic application of the ideas presented. As Kurt Lewin has argued, there is nothing as practical as a good theory.

The first four chapters focus on interpersonal interaction. All four begin with the assumption that the choices individuals make about safer sex practices only can be understood through an examination of the communication dynamics surrounding sexual intercourse. Metts and Fitzpatrick (chapter 1) illustrate the embedded and dynamic nature of condom use by situating it within a cognitive model based on scripts and plans. Although speculative, the model presumes that the prevailing sexual script warrants against condom use. Next, Kashima, Gallois, and McCamish (chapter 2) employ Fishbein and Ajzen's Theory of Reasoned Action to explore the role of peer norms in sexual decision making. They present data collected from heterosexual and homosexual populations in Australia to highlight the relationship between social influences and the negotiation of safer sex practices. Edgar (chapter 3) focuses on the function of influence strategies in the use of condoms. He uses Dillard's Goals-Planning-Action model of compliance gaining as a guide to show how the perception of one's own communicative resources affects the ability to develop and enact plans for sexual interaction. Adelman (chapter 4) argues that the notion of safer sex represents a psychologically incongruent frame and demonstrates how the metaphor of negotiation is limited for understanding the reconciliation of this incongruity. She relies on theories of play and humor to illustrate how alternative views of the process may contribute to the facilitation of safer sexual encounters. The next three chapters concentrate on issues relevant to public campaigns about AIDS. Freimuth (chapter 5) begins with a general overview of typologies of theories useful for AIDS campaigns and describes applications of selected theories. The following two chapters describe specific campaigns on two different continents. Marková and Power (chapter 6) spotlight educational efforts in the United Kingdom. They show how social representations (i.e., collectively formed and maintained explanations for human activities) mold the environment within which people think about and conceptualize AIDS-related phenomena and how these phenomena have a powerful effect on the individual. Salmon and Kroger (chapter 7) adopt a systems theory framework for describing the National AIDS Information and Education Program, a federally funded, multifaceted national system charged with educating the "general public" in the United States about AIDS. The Michal-Johnson and Bowen chapter (8) on intercultural issues encompasses problems of interpersonal communication as well as concerns about public campaigns. They argue that culture contextualizes people's understanding of health and illness and affects how they respond through communicative actions. The final two chapters are devoted to the ways in which AIDS has been treated by the news media. Dearing and Rogers (chapter 9) utilize the concept of agenda setting to identify the main factors that influenced the importance of AIDS as a newsworthy issue in San Francisco and in the United States as a whole. McAllister (chapter 10) ends with a critical approach toward understanding news coverage of AIDS. He explores the "Medicalization of Society" thesis as a theoretical approach to understanding the expansive and political nature of Western medicine.

ACKNOWLEDGMENTS

We wish to thank our contributors who have been a model group. We appreciated the manner in which they continually met our deadlines (or at least came close), and we valued their openness to our feedback throughout the editorial process. Finally, we extend special thanks to Courtney Plotnick for her many hours of editorial assistance and to Glenn Fleischman for his help with the index.

Timothy Edgar
Mary Anne Fitzpatrick
Vicki S. Freimuth

CHAPTER ONE

Thinking About Safer Sex: The Risky Business of "Know Your Partner" Advice

Sandra Metts
Illinois State University

Mary Anne Fitzpatrick
University of Wisconsin

Despite repeated media warnings about the association between "unprotected sex" and AIDS transmission, major national samples indicate that consistent use of condoms is not a typical practice for large numbers of sexually active persons, especially within the heterosexual population (Catania et al., 1989). One often voiced barrier to condom use is a negative attitude toward condoms (e.g., reduced sensitivity, loss of spontaneity during intercourse, discomfort, unpleasant odor, and messiness; Sonnex, Hart, Williams, & Adler, 1989). A more psychological obstacle is the fact that the onset of the disease may be delayed for up to 7 years or more following exposure to the virus. Thus, the immediate consequences of sexual activity are reinforcing, whereas the negative consequences of unprotected sex are uncertain and removed in time from the sexual act (Kelly, St. Lawrence, Hood, & Brasfield, 1989).

It is misleading however to assume that all people who engage in sexual intercourse without using condoms are unaware of or have flagrant disregard for safer-sex practices. Many sexually active people do not use condoms but assume they engage in safer sex because they have intercourse only with persons they believe to be "safe." Interviews with heterosexual college students revealed that the "most popular prophylactic" was the selection of a noninfected sexual partner (Maticka-Tyndale, 1991). Confidence in the safe partner strategy among this group was fostered by two presumptions. First, because sexual partners are typically chosen from a group of friends within the social network, they are presumed

1

to be trustworthy and safe, and second, because "unsafe" people are presumed to be somehow distinguishable from safe people, they can be recognized and avoided as sexual partners. This suggests that the female college student who would never meet a stranger in a bar and engage in unprotected intercourse with him is highly likely to meet her roommate's brother and feel that insistence on using a condom is not necessary.

Remarkably, even when education is directed toward careful delineation of safer-sex practices, partner selection persists as the preferred strategy. After a 10-week university course on human sexuality, Baldwin, Whiteley, and Baldwin (1990) found that course students (compared to a control group) worried more about AIDS, became more "selective" about partners, and asked more questions of partners about AIDS-related behavior. However, these students did not increase their use of condoms, decrease their number of sexual partners, nor spend a longer time getting to know new partners before engaging in sexual activity. Prevention efforts may simply work to increase naive information-seeking behavior rather than foster positive behavioral changes.

Belief in the ability to select a "safe partner" as the preferred method of safer sex may not be medically sound, but it is consistent with what would be expected from persons trying to cope with multiple, often competing goals (see, e.g., O'Keefe, 1991). Because sexual experience is embedded in a larger web of relational, social, and cultural forces, practicing safer sex through condom use is an enormously complicated endeavor. Achieving that goal often creates tension as it crosses the goals of other concerns such as the desire to avoid face threat, embarrassment, and relational strain.

The purpose of this chapter is to illustrate the embedded and dynamic nature of condom use by situating it within a cognitive model based on scripts and plans. Although speculative, the model presumes that the prevailing sexual script warrants against condom use because condoms disrupt the passion of the moment, they signify ghosts of lovers past, and particularly because they symbolize the possibility that one or both partners are infected with the AIDS virus. Thus, although the prevailing script does include a "getting to know each other" phase that allows for explicit questions about a potential partner's use of condoms, the pressure to be socially appropriate leads people to assess less relevant features of a target—typically his or her suitability as a relational (rather than sexual) partner (Cline, Freeman, Johnson, 1990; Edgar, Freimuth, Hammond, McDonald, & Fink, in press). Relatively few individuals progress through the subsequent phases that request or demand the use of a condom. Indeed, even beginning the sexual encounter with the idea that alternatives to condom usage are possible mitigates against the final decision to use a condom.

The model also recognizes, however, creative and flexible variations within the constraints of the generalized sexual script. These variations are goal-directed action sequences, or plans. Sexually active people who have plans for achieving the goal of condom use seek information from potential partners that help them effectively introduce and gain compliance for condom use. We would expect, therefore, that communication in the "getting to know each other" phase for these people differs in important ways from the communication of partners using more scripted routines.

A PHENOMENOLOGICAL DEFINITION OF SAFER SEX

The statistical probability of contacting AIDS through sexual activity can be reduced by abstaining from sexual activity entirely, avoiding sexual activity with high-risk partners (e.g., homosexual/bisexual males, intravenous drug users, and persons with multiple partners), limiting the number of sexual partners, avoiding receptive anal intercourse, and using condoms. Among the findings of importance in comparing these methods is that using condoms is the most effective preventive measure for sexually active people. Reiss and Leik (1989) utilized probability modeling to test the risk reduction value of two of the behavioral strategies: decreasing the number of sexual partners and using condoms. Their results indicated that "consistent and careful condom use is a far more effective method of reducing HIV infection" (p. 411) than is reducing the number of sexual partners.

Some researchers have argued that condoms are infrequently used because of the negative beliefs that men and women have about condoms (Hebert, Bernard, de Man, & Farrar, 1989; Sonnex et al., 1989). Although the development of intervention programs to change these negative beliefs should continue (e.g., Cohen, Dent, & MacKinnon, 1991), a largely unexplored facet of condom usage in heterosexual intercourse involves the *reproductive* and *relational* significance associated with condoms.

Among heterosexuals, condoms are considered a method for birth control rather than a means for preventing sexually transmitted diseases (STDs; Maticka-Tyndale, 1991; Sonnex et al., 1989). Thus, sexually active couples tend to use other forms of contraception (typically birth control pills), reducing the risk of pregnancy but increasing the risk of exposure to AIDS.

Moreover, even when condoms are recognized for their protective function against STDs, they are used primarily during early or casual sexual episodes. Condoms tend to be abandoned once a relationship develops some degree of commitment and trust. Even prostitutes, who consistently use condoms with their clients, will signify that their private relationship is "special" by not using condoms during sexual activity (Des Jarlais & Friedman, 1988; Maticka-Tyndale, 1991). Continued use of condoms in a developed relationship, especially when other methods of birth control are being used, seems to represent distance/formality rather than intimacy, or may suggest that infidelity is present or suspected (Fullilove, Fullilove, Haynes, & Gross, 1990; Mays & Cochran, 1988). Thus, what condoms mean to relative strangers is not what they mean to relational partners.

Given the negative beliefs about condoms and the shifting meaning of condoms depending on the nature of the interpersonal relationship between sexual partners, the default strategy for most sexually active individuals is to avoid sexual activity with high-risk partners. In a brochure on AIDS mailed to every American household by the Surgeon General's office in 1988, readers were told that if you knew another person well enough to have sex with him or her, then you had a responsibility to ask that person questions about his or her background. The brochure suggested asking: Had the partner ever had any sexually transmitted disease? Did the partner ever experiment with drugs? How many people has the partner been to bed with? These questions are designed to help the information processor evaluate the risk of having unprotected intercourse with a partner.

Survey studies indicate that individuals do not ask these questions. A survey of 459 college students indicated that only 27% were likely to ask a new sexual partner how many previous sexual partners he or she had been involved with, whereas 60% were likely to "try to guess" if a new partner had been exposed to AIDS (Gray & Saracino, 1991). Edgar et al. (in press) found that approximately 75% of their sample of sexually active college men and women (N = 204) were not confident that they knew the number of people their partners had been to bed with and about 43% were only moderately confident about whether their partner had ever had a sexually transmitted disease. Despite these concerns, more than half (57%) engaged in unprotected intercourse anyway.

In the next section, we offer a model of sexual communication used by most individuals who from their own phenomenological point of view are heeding the warning to know their partner as a way to practice safer sex.

A COGNITIVE PERSPECTIVE
ON SEXUAL COMMUNICATION

In this section, we argue that most individuals follow relatively scripted behavior in sexual encounters. This behavior specifies that information-seeking strategies be deployed to confirm assumptions that a potential sexual partner is "safe." The scripted nature of these behaviors tend to preclude judgments that a partner is "risky." If such evaluations were made, the information processor would be placed in the position of requesting a partner to use a condom. To the extent that the prevailing sexual script does not prepare individuals very well for this contingency, they may find themselves limited to two options: having unprotected sex or abstaining from sexual intercourse with that partner.

Within this section, we also discuss the fact that some individuals move beyond scripted routines and seem to anticipate and be prepared for this contingency. Indeed, they have highly complex and abstract plans to insure condom use, both when the suggestion is readily accepted by the partner and when it is resisted. These "planners" have a different initial information-seeking strategy in that the goal is to assess the beliefs and attitudes of a potential partner toward condoms in the interest of developing a "successful" plan to incorporate condoms as part of the sexual episode.

Sexual Scripts

According to Simon and Gagnon (1987), sexual behavior is influenced by three types of scripts: the cultural, the interpersonal, and the intrapsychic. The cultural script grows out of the scenarios presented in the media, folklore, and mythology that "instruct" cultural members in appropriate goals, desirable qualities, and typical behaviors for sexual and potentially sexual experiences. Interpersonal scripts contain interactional strategies designed to accomplish sexual encounters with specific others. Such strategies are individually implemented but derived from an understanding of what cultural scenarios depict. Intraphysic scripts are idiosyncratic "maps" of the motives and reasons for an individual's sexual behavior. They enable a person to link individual sexual desires, arousal, eroticism, and fantasy to social meaning.

Sexual scripts, then, provide a basis for generating, anticipating, and interpreting primarily routinized and/or role-defined sexual behavior. Scripts provide little instruction, however, for appropriate behavioral sequences in novel, ambiguous, and emergent situations—precisely the kind of situation in which sexually active people find themselves when they want to have sex with an unfamiliar sexual partner.

Evidence of the lack of specificity in the scripts for safer-sex episodes is available in a series of studies performed by Edgar and Fitzpatrick (1991). In the first study, participants were asked to describe an "evening" that would lead to and include sexual intercourse. These descriptions revealed well-developed scripts for the "romance" part of the evening (e.g., "they dance," "he compliments her," "she smiles coyly"). The detail and number of sequences diminished, however, when the episode became explicitly sexual and yielded simple, inclusive phrases (e.g., "they practice safer sex"). No respondent spontaneously mentioned asking a partner any of the questions related to risk factors and condom use before having intercourse. In a second study, subjects were asked to rate the degree to which these various behaviors were typical and necessary. Even though "practicing safer sex" was a segment of the script that received very high ratings on necessity, it received very low ratings on typicality. This stands in contrast to the ratings for sequences such as "female smiles coyly," which received low necessity ratings, but high typicality ratings.

The two broad phases of what we have termed the *prevailing sexual script* are presented here. The first is labeled the information-seeking phase and the second is labeled the express/request condom phase.

Information-Seeking Phase

Efforts to learn as much as possible as quickly as possible about a person to whom we are attracted is not a condition unique to sexual scripts. Uncertainty about other people in social situations is an uncomfortable state and we generally seek to reduce it. Although uncertainty is a function of both the ability to predict and the ability to explain behavior, individuals typically obtain information that increases their predictive certainty before they become concerned with explaining why certain behaviors have (or have not) occurred. Thus, the prevailing sexual script would suggest that persons who are unfamiliar with each other (or even perhaps who are familiar with each other) would attempt to gather information ("know your partner") that would confirm their initial predictions that a potential sexual partner was safe.

Uncertainty is reduced through the use of passive, active, and interactive strategies (Berger, 1987a; Berger & Bradac, 1982). Passive strategies allow observers to gain information about others by observing them without their knowledge. Active strategies require the observer to do something to affect the response of the actor, without actually having any direct contact. Interactive strategies involve face-to-face interaction between the observer and the actor. In Table 1.1, we list the possible tactics under the information-seeking strategies.

Given the potential face threat of seeking sexual histories and attitudes toward condoms, we might expect individuals to prefer the more indirect strategies. However, this seems not to be the case (Edgar et al., in press), probably because they are highly inefficient. The passive strategies would require far too many instances of observation in order to reliably decide about the "safety" of a partner. And, even if an observer could decide that a given partner was in all probability neither promiscuous nor an

TABLE 1.1
Knowing Your Partner

Passive Strategies

1. Reactivity search—Observe target in a social situation where he or she is "active"
   Example: How does she respond during conversations with other people?
2. Disinhibition search—Observe target in informal situations where constraints (inhibitions) are lowered
   Example: Does he display more aggressive behavior when drinking alcohol than when at work?

Active Strategies

1. Ask others about target—Uses members of the social network and network gossip to gain information about target
   Example: Does she sleep around?
2. Environmental structuring—Manipulates some aspect of physical or social environment to see how target reacts
   Example: Have a friend "come on" to a target to see how he or she responds.

Interactive Strategies

1. Self-disclosure—Giving personal information (in anticipation that target will reciprocate)
   Example: I am really afraid about AIDS.
2. Interrogation—Asking questions directly to target
   Example: Have you been tested? May I see the results?

Adapted from Berger and Bradac (1982).

intravenous drug user, the information processor could still not examine all of a given individual's previous partners.

The active strategies are somewhat more efficient, although the information processor does not know whether or not the target has been informed of the questions and, of course, the veracity of gossip, in general, is questionable. The ability to actually structure a physical or social situation in order to see the reaction of another communicator is also open to question. Few social scientists are themselves very good at structuring experimental situations on either a physical or social dimension to reveal, unambiguously, the probability of a given human behavior or trait.

The interactive strategies are the most direct means of gaining information about a potential partner. Given the serious consequences of contacting AIDS, we might predict that interrogation (explicit questions about sexual history and intentions regarding use of condoms) would be the predominant tactic, in spite of its possible face threat. The prevailing script, however, seems to favor more generalized and unfocused discussions of "safer sex," at least during initial interactions between heterosexual couples (Caron, Bertran, & McMullen, 1987). Even in relationships characterized by sexual frequency and/or exclusivity, talk about AIDS and safer sex may not be common. Surveys asking couples whether they "have ever discussed AIDS" (e.g., Sprecher, 1990) yield high numbers, often almost three quarters of the sample. The talk, however, is not concrete but rather abstract, and focuses on relationships in general and not on the emerging relationship. Cline et al. (1990) surveyed a large heterosexual college population concerning their level of talk about safer sex. They found that about 21% had discussed safer sex with their sexual partner ("safe-sex talkers"), including AIDS prevention, condom use, sexual history, or monogamy. However, 80% had either discussed AIDS-related topics out of the context of their personal relationship or had never discussed AIDS with a partner at all.

To some degree the lack of focused, partner-specific discussion can be attributed to a feeling of invulnerability with regards to contracting AIDS. This is especially true in the heterosexual population, the college student population, and among males (Baldwin & Baldwin, 1988; Hansen, Hahn, & Wolkenstein, 1990).

It is also true, however, that directness in information gathering is associated with judgments of reduced social appropriateness (Berger & Kellerman, 1983). This leaves the information seeker in a dilemma. High levels of uncertainty about important issues strongly encourages efficient information-gaining strategies because these are associated with attributional confidence. However, efficient strategies (direct questions) may result in decreased attraction. To be unattractive is to inhibit reaching the goal of most dating encounters: the development of a romantic relationship. In response, there seems to have emerged an interpretive bias in the prevailing sexual script toward assessing any willingness to discuss sex as "evidence" that this person is a safe partner and trustworthy.

Information seekers apparently take their partners' willingness to talk about AIDS, in any fashion, as evidence of honesty and openness and thereby attribute lesser risk to that partner (Cline et al., 1990). The most obvious flaw in this assumption is that people are often ignorant about their own sexual history and are often not honest. Cochran and Mays (1990) asked 422 sexually active college students if they had told a lie in order to have sex. Thirty-four percent of the men and 10% of the women said they had lied to have sex. Sixty-eight percent of the men and 59% of the women said they have been involved with more than one person and their partner did not know. When asked whether they had been lied to by a partner, 47% of the men and 60% of the women said their partner had lied to them to have sex.

Exit or Continue. Those individuals whose uncertainty has been replaced by confidence that they have selected a safe partner will exit the model at this point (have unprotected sex), unless their partner expresses the desire to use a condom. To the extent that such a request is surprising (prompts new levels of uncertainty), they may reengage information-seeking strategies. Those individuals whose uncertainty has been replaced by confidence that they have selected an unsafe partner may also exit the model at this point (no sex), unless the desire to have sex and/or confidence in the preventive utility of condoms motivates them to continue to the second phase of the model.

Another group of individuals may exit at this point because they are unwilling or unable to enact the next phase. They simply cannot perform the action sequences necessary to raise the issue of using a condom (see Edgar, this volume; Zimmerman, 1989). And the entire information-seeking phase was designed to find out that the partner was safe, so un-covering information that the partner may be a risky choice places the communicator in a difficult position. Fairly late in the sequence, he or she is going into a request-to-use-a-condom phase with little information on the partner's views on that issue. Exit from the model will as likely be manifested as unprotected sex as no sex.

Express/Request Phase

Expressing one's desire to use a condom or requesting that one's part-ner use a condom is inherently face threatening. This is especially the case when the encounter has been proceeding along an information-seeking trajectory. It is very clear to both communicators that some un-pleasant information has been uncovered or condoms would not now be the focus of the exchange.

By its very nature, expressing the desire to use a condom is an implicit disclosure of fear and anxiety about AIDS, fears that have not been al-layed during the information-seeking phase. One may believe that to ex-press these anxieties openly exposes one's negative (possibly promiscuous) self and increases the possibility of rejection by a potential partner. An individual also might feel that insistence on condom usage may be con-strued as an insult by the other person. The revelation of one's feelings about taking preventive measures can communicate tacitly a suspicion that one's partner is infected with the AIDS virus. If an individual is very sensitive about forming a positive impression, then he or she is likely to avoid the communication of any messages that might call into question the partner's character or behavior.

Although very little research has been done on how partners actually request that condoms be used, we can formulate a general structure for the plan by drawing on politeness theory (Brown & Levinson, 1987). To the extent that introducing condoms is face threatening, partners will likely sacrifice efficiency in favor of appropriateness, at least initially.

Thus, the episode will be marked by indirectness—a strong preference that yields only slowly to directness. This characterization would be consistent with patterns found in other sequences during the negotiation of sexual intercourse, all of which tend to be characterized by a norm of indirectness, implicature, and ambiguity (Jesser, 1978; McCormick, 1987; McCormick & Jesser, 1983; Perper & Weis, 1987).

Politeness theory posits that people have positive face needs (the desire to be appreciated and approved of) and negative face needs (the desire to be free from imposition and restraint) (Brown & Levinson, 1987). Many social actions (e.g., requests, complaints, rejections) are face threatening. Five strategies for dealing with the inevitability of face threat, from least to most face threatening and most to least efficient, are: (a) bald on record without redressive action, (b) on record with positive politeness, (c) on record with negative politeness, (d) off record/hint, (e) not do the face threatening act.

Requesting that a condom be used during intercourse threatens the requestor's positive face and the positive face of the partner in the implication that one or both might carry the HIV virus. Like any request, it also threatens the negative face of the partner in that it impedes or constrains that person's behavior. Although hinting and other off-record strategies are not very efficient, they are more face preserving than going on record. Thus, hinting is a logical first-level strategy. If the hint works, face threat has been minimal and the overt move to introduce the condom will then originate with the partner.

A similar pattern is found in an analogous sequence, sexual rejection. Although expressing the desire to use a condom is not a rejection message, it can be perceived as a delay tactic similar to the first message in a rejection sequence (Metts, Cupach, & Imahori, 1992). Rejecting a sexual overture and requesting condom use are both problematic in that the metagoals of efficiency and appropriateness are competing. Both use indirectness as a mechanism to resolve the tension. For example, both of the general categories of behaviors designed to resist sexual involvement identified by Perper and Weis (1987) in the essays of college females are indirect: avoid receptivity (e.g., avoiding intimate situations and ignoring sexual advances) and incomplete rejection (e.g., remaining affectionate but hinting for the pursuer to stop). This preference for indirectness becomes even more pronounced (among female subjects) when the rejector is romantically interested in an insistent partner (Byers & Lewis, 1988). It is reasonable to assume a similar trend for expressing the desire to use a condom.

If, however, the partner does not recognize the hint, or prefers not to comply, the person desiring to use a condom must go "on record" with more direct requests. In so doing, the requestor is more likely to redress the face of his or her partner with positive and negative politeness than to go "bald on record" and request the use of a condom without an account.

We would expect from the accounts literature that requestors would justify their request in ways that address partner's face. For example, we might expect a woman who requests that her male partner use a condom would provide, perhaps, "fear of pregnancy" as an explanation rather than "fear of AIDS." This excuse might be used even in situations where the female requestor is protected by birth control pills. In most cultures, the implication that a man could make a woman pregnant is more face preserving than the implication that he could give her AIDS. And within a traditional female script, not being on the birth control pill is proof that one was swept away by the moment rather than that one planned to have intercourse.

Exit or Continue.   Most individuals will exit the model at this point (have safer sex) if the request to use a condom is met with a positive response from a willing partner. We predict that some individuals will exit the model at this point (have unprotected sex) if the request is met with a negative response and competing goals are more important (e.g., to preserve the relationship, or have sex under any circumstances).

A much smaller percentage of individuals will exit the model at this point (abstain) if the partner resists the request and (a) the goal of having intercourse is relatively unimportant (not worth additional investment of time or the risk of infection) or (b) the requestor feels incompetent gaining compliance because they lack highly detailed and developed contingent plans (Berger, 1988).

An even smaller percentage of individuals will stay in the model and move to the next phase where strategies are used to gain compliance from a reluctant partner (see Edgar, this volume).

Summary

In this section, we have discussed what we believe to be the more common scripted route taken by individuals who practice safer sex. The information-seeking phase functions primarily to confirm the suitability of a prospective partner. In the unfolding of interaction between partners, strategies are devised in order to support the hypothesis that the partner is not a risk. Numerous studies have demonstrated that in collecting social information, we find the answer we seek (e.g., Snyder & Campbell, 1980). The phase of requesting that a condom be used is far less likely to be entered and when the decision is made to do so, it is seldom based on information gained during the previous phase. This phase tends to follow norms of indirectness and ambiguity and is easily derailed if the condom is resisted at its first mention.

In the next section, we briefly discuss an alternative scenario in which certain individuals have highly developed plans for using condoms that start in an information-seeking phase designed not to discover that the partner is safe but rather to discover the partner's attitudes toward condoms. Plans differ from scripts in that they are generated strategically in pursuit of a specific goal (Berger, 1988). Less routinized, plans enable actors to perform in novel, ambiguous, and dynamic episodes such as negotiating condom usage in sexual encounters.

PLANS TO USE CONDOMS

Some couples do use condoms and do so with little or no disruption to the sexual episode or the relationship. This accomplishment suggests that individuals are able to generate, coordinate, and enact plans for using condoms (Metts & Cupach, 1991). Moreover, the most successful plans seem to allow for maximum efficiency (i.e., minimal disruption to the "romantic" tenor of the moment) and maximum appropriateness (i.e., minimum risk to the face of self and partner and minimum damage to the perceived specialness of the relationship). As we argue, however, those who use condoms in sexual encounters start with flexible and dynamic plans directed, from the beginning of the encounter, toward the goal of using a condom if intercourse takes place.

Unfortunately, we know little about the overall structure and contingency moves of successful plans (see Berger, 1987b, for an example of a date request plan) or how successful condom planners generate and enact plans. To date, research efforts have been limited to describing tactics and strategies for gaining compliance with the request to use condoms (e.g., Edgar & Fitzpatrick, 1988; Metts & Cupach, 1991). The way contingency actions are mapped onto primary actions and revised when elements of the episode change has not yet been uncovered. Certainly the scientific observation of intimate interaction is problematic, but creative use of role-play techniques should facilitate the process (e.g., Adelman, 1991).

This caveat aside, however, we can offer what we know to be influences on the ability to generate successful plans. We begin with the unfortunate paradox that heterosexual women are by far the most in need of successful plans for condom use, but also the most likely to be paralyzed by the prevailing sexual script.

Gender-Role Constraints

Condom use in heterosexual couples cannot be considered apart from gender and gender-role expectations. Survey data indicate that women are more likely than men to report having discussed safer sex with their sexual partner (24% vs. 17%), and to have had general discussions about AIDS outside the context of their relationship (48% vs. 37%; Cline et al., 1990). This openness may be due primarily to the more extensive education females receive in health and personal safety (Baldwin et al., 1990). Women also learn early that most consequences of sexual activities are more costly to them than to males, both in terms of unwanted pregnancies and undesirable reputations. Thus, women tend to be more active in assessing the emotional and sexual climate of a relationship. This awareness does not necessarily empower women, however, to be more effective in accomplishing safer sex.

Men are less likely than women to report having talked about AIDS at all (24% vs. 41%; Cline et al., 1990). Men report feeling less vulnerable to the HIV infection than do women (Hansen et al., 1990) and report stronger negative reactions to condoms. These patterns are exaggerated in cultures where concern for AIDS and interest in condom use are considered not machismo. Some cultures and ethnic groups place a value on risk and some men do not want to appear less risky than their peers.

Two groups of women are particularly disadvantaged in the development of plans to use condoms: (a) women who have internalized the traditional gender-role script and (b) women who must negotiate from a position of powerlessness relative to their relationship partner.

The traditional gender-role script defines the male role as sexually assertive and experienced, a lover who initiates the shy and inexperienced female to her first sexual experience (Komarovsky, 1976; Laws & Schwartz, 1977). If a woman endorses the traditional gender role, she is in a very difficult position in terms of insisting that her partner use a condom. On the one hand, she is at great risk with a sexually experienced partner. But on the other hand, forthright and determined arguments are inconsistent with sexual naivete and may imply sexual promiscuity to a traditional male partner or to a male partner whose culture places value on female virginity (e.g., Hispanic). Moreover, the vocabulary available to women for discussing sex is less varied and more clinical than the vocabulary available to men (Kutner & Brogan, 1974; Sanders & Robinson, 1979). Thus, a woman may feel limited in the ability to be assertive about her safer-sex preferences and limited in the linguistic resources to communicate her preferences in an erotic manner.

Women who are sexually experienced and/or do not subscribe to the traditional gender-role script will exert more explicit control of the situation. Grauerholtz and Serpe (1985) found that the more sexually liberal a woman is in terms of instructing her partner, masturbating, and the greater her number of sexual partners, the more likely she is to exercise proactive sexual moves. Thus, the extent to which a woman subscribes to the traditional gender-role script will, in part, determine the extent to which she allows concerns other than the risk of AIDS to determine her insistence on using condoms.

Women who enter the sexual arena with little power relative to their partner will also find that insisting on condom use is difficult to do. Although women can feel powerless for many reasons, a common origin is in gender ratios that favor men (e.g., in the Hispanic, African-American, and elderly communities). The number of potential male partners who can provide stable and enduring relationships is smaller than the number of women who are seeking such a relationship (Fullilove et al., 1990). As a result, women are simply less likely to insist on condom use during intercourse as a criterion for remaining in the relationship. There are many other women available who will not, and are therefore more attractive to a reluctant partner.

Researchers often have a difficult time considering any research participant as an "expert." Yet, rather than focusing our energies on college age men and women who are not using condoms, we need to go to samples of sexually experienced individuals and examine in great detail the strategies these successful planners use to get partners, even reluctant ones, to use condoms. Of particular focus are sexually expert women who have highly detailed plans. Research needs to focus on these plans and how they are developed and instantiated and how these women meet resistance. It may be that sexually expert women negotiate condom usage long before the actual sexual encounter. We suspect that sexually expert women spend the time used by others in ineffective information seeking to probe for potential resistance to condom usage on the part of the male partner.

Research into how to make the passive and active information-seeking strategies used by naive or traditional women into more effective tools may be necessary. For example, in cultures where women are negatively sanctioned for being sexually experienced but where women have strong social networks, these networks may be used more effectively to help women to find out information about risky partners before they even engage in interaction, let alone intercourse, with them.

Summary

We have argued that both males and females follow relatively scripted sexual communication scenarios and that the prevention of AIDS is seriously hampered by these scripts. Operating with preexisting scripts, men and women conduct ineffective information searches to determine the riskiness of a partner. The number of individuals who have highly detailed and elaborated plans for using condoms in sexual encounters is probably small yet worth extensive investigation. Because the onus differentially falls on women, we believe that studies should concentrate on how sexually active and independent women structure goal-oriented sequences to insure that condoms are used in sexual encounters. In addition, we believe that studies examining a greater use of passive and active information-seeking strategies be undertaken to give women with less power more help in deciding risk. In the conclusion of this chapter, we discuss the implications of our cognitive model for primary prevention.

IMPLICATIONS FOR PREVENTION

Although this chapter is not intended to provide a comprehensive prevention program, the problems that we believe to be endemic to the prevailing sexual script suggest two areas for attention. First, the notion that a "safe partner" can be recognized through skillful information seeking must be disallowed. Sexually active people must be cautioned that condoms are always advisable, despite argument to the contrary from partners and despite confidence in their perceptions of partners. Educational messages must emphasize that selecting safe partners as an adequate protection against HIV is based on a probability calculation. Unfortunately, a person's history of risk behaviors is difficult to know completely. "You know if you're using a condom or you're not. You don't know if you're picking the right partner" ("Heterosexual AIDS," 1988).

Although documentaries and media coverage that show AIDS patients near death have done a great deal to increase sympathy for the victims and increase America's awareness of the seriousness of the disease, they have possibly contributed to the "I can recognize an unsafe partner" belief. Media coverage of persons who are HIV positive, but who are attempting to conduct their lives in a "normal" fashion would remind the public that carriers of HIV do not indicate their status in any observable way.

Second, prevention efforts must be directed more systematically toward communication training. It cannot be assumed that sexual communication competence is learned in school or from peer groups. Although information about AIDS and condom use is presented in most sex education courses, the focus is on facts rather than the pragmatics of achieving sexual communication competence (Adelman, 1989; D'Augelli & D'Augelli, 1985). Little or no attention is given to communication techniques for managing competing goals or for enacting information-seeking episodes that lead smoothly to and through protected sexual involvement.

Faulty information-processing strategies based on the assumption that safe partners can be isolated must be replaced with information-processing strategies designed to elicit the partner's views about condoms, and alternative sexual practices that might be employed if condoms are not used. This is not to imply that efforts to increase awareness and increase perceptions of risk should be abandoned, only that they must be augmented with programs responsive to the interactive, relational, and cultural environment that influence the probability of condom use.

Even the media, a dependable source for depicting at least some version of a culture's sexual script, have not addressed the issue of how couples negotiate condom use. Larson (1991) analyzed the treatment of the AIDS issue when the soap opera "All My Children" ran a storyline involving two characters who were in danger of contracting or had contracted the disease. Characters (and real-life experts) discussed how the disease was transmitted, how testing was performed, and how prejudice/ignorance about the disease was perpetuated. But the prevention of AIDS was not discussed by sexually active couples, some of whom had multiple partners. One television program that has explicitly included condoms in depictions of sexual episodes is an adult comedy called "Dream On." The efforts here are to be applauded for their innovation. Unfortunately, the characters who use condoms all agree—without dialogue—that condoms are essential. A viewer whose partner was not well educated, not middle class, and not favorably disposed toward condoms would still have no communication interactions to emulate.

It is not likely that public television and film will include explicit portrayals of couples negotiating condom use; it is not yet part of the romantic abandon and unbridled passion that has come to characterize the Western romantic myth. However, it would be possible for public media to include conversations among members of the social network about condoms and the messages that were used to encourage condom use with resistant partners.

Finally, communication training should not be limited to individuals and casual daters but should include established couples as well. Because couples often abandon condoms once they feel committed and exclusive, instruction should be aimed at reconceptualizing condoms. Relationships are a web of attributions and actions that give meaning to sexual acts. To discontinue using condoms may represent an intensification move for the couple, but it does not constitute protection. Skills in communicating about the relationship and the meaning of sex acts in the relationship reduce uncertainty and enhance overall relational satisfaction.

REFERENCES

Adelman, M. B. (1989, May). *Safe-sex talk: Curriculum for course instruction.* Paper presented at the Iowa Conference on Personal and Social Relationships, Iowa City, IA.

Adelman, M. B. (1991). Play and incongruity: Framing safe-sex talk. *Health Communication, 3,* 139–155.

Baldwin, J. D., & Baldwin, J. I. (1988). Factors affecting AIDS-related sexual risk-taking behavior among college students. *Journal of Sex Research, 25,* 181–196.

Baldwin, J. I., Whiteley, S., & Baldwin, J. D. (1990). Changing AIDS- and fertility-related behavior: The effectiveness of sexual education. *Journal of Sex Research, 27,* 245–262.

Berger, C. R. (1987a). Communicating under uncertainty. In M. E. Roloff & G. R. Miller (Eds.), *Interpersonal processes: New directions in communication research* (pp. 39–62). Newbury Park, CA: Sage.

Berger, C. R. (1987b). Planning and scheming: Strategies for initiating relationships. In R. Burnett, P. McGhee, & D. Clarke (Eds.), *Accounting for relationships: Explanation, representation and knowledge* (pp. 158–174). London: Methuen.

Berger, C. R. (1988). Planning, affect, and social action generation. In L. Donohew, H. E. Sypher, & E. T. Higgins (Eds.), *Communication, social cognition, and affect* (pp. 93–116). Hillsdale, NJ: Lawrence Erlbaum Associates.

Berger, C. R., & Bradac, J. J. (1982). *Language and social knowledge: Uncertainty in interpersonal relationships.* London: Edward Arnold.

Berger, C., & Kellermann, K. (1983). To ask or not to ask: Is that a question? In R. N. Bostrom (Ed.), *Communication yearbook 7* (pp. 342–368). Newbury Park, CA: Sage.

Brown, P., & Levinson, S. C. (1987). *Politeness: Some universals in language use.* Cambridge: Cambridge University Press.

Byers, E. S., & Lewis, K. (1988). Dating couples' disagreements over the desired level of sexual intimacy. *Journal of Sex Research, 24,* 15–29.

Caron, S. L., Bertran, R. M., & McMullen, T. (1987). AIDS and the college student: The need for sex education. *SIECUS Report, 15*(6), 6–7.

Catania, J. A., Coates, T. J., Greenblatt, R. M., Dolcini, M. M., Kegeles, S. M., Puckett, S., Corman, M., & Miller, J. (1989). Predictors of condom use and multiple partnered sex among sexually active adolescent women: Implications for AIDS-related health interventions. *Journal of Sex Research, 4,* 514–524.

Cline, R. J. W., Freeman, K. E., & Johnson, S. J. (1990). Talk among sexual partners about AIDS: Factors differentiating those who talk from those who do not. *Communication Research, 17,* 792–808.

Cochran, S. D., & Mays, V. M. (1990). Sex, lies, and HIV. *New England Journal of Medicine, 322,* 774–775.

Cohen, D., Dent, C., & MacKinnon, D. (1991). Condom skills education and sexually transmitted disease reinfection. *Journal of Sex Research, 28,* 139–144.

D'Augelli, A., & D'Augelli, J. F. (1985). The enhancement of sexual skills and competence. In L. L'Abate & M. A. Milan (Eds.), *Handbook of social skills training and research* (pp. 170–191). New York: Wiley.

Des Jarlais, D. C., & Friedman, S. R. (1988). The psychology of preventing AIDS among intravenous drug users: A social learning conceptualization. *American Psychologist, 43,* 865–870.

Edgar, T., & Fitzpatrick, M. A. (1988). Compliance-gaining in relational interaction: When your life depends on it. *Southern Speech Communication Journal, 53,* 385–405.

Edgar, T., & Fitzpatrick, M. A. (1991). *Memory structures for sexual interaction: A cognitive test of the sequencing of sexual communication behaviors.* Manuscript submitted for publication.

Edgar, T., Freimuth, V. S., Hammond, S. L., McDonald, D. A., & Fink, E. L. (in press). Strategic sexual communication: Condom use resistance and response. *Health Communication.*

Fullilove, M. T., Fullilove, R. E., Haynes, K., & Gross, S. (1990). Black women and AIDS prevention: A view towards understanding the gender rules. *Journal of Sex Research, 27,* 47–64.

Grauerholz, E., & Serpe, R. T. (1985). Initiation and response: The dynamics of sexual interaction. *Sex Roles, 12,* 1041–1059.

Gray, L. A., & Saracino, M. (1991). College students' attitudes, beliefs, and behaviors about AIDS: Implications for family life educators. *Family Relations, 40,* 258–263.

Hansen, W. B., Hahn, G. L., & Wolkenstein, B. H. (1990). Perceived personal immunity: Beliefs about susceptibility to AIDS. *Journal of Sex Research, 27,* 622–628.

Hebert, Y., Bernard, J., de Man, A. F., & Farrar, D. (1989). Factors related to the use of condoms among French-Canadian university students. *Journal of Social Psychology, 129,* 707–709.

Heterosexual AIDS: Setting the odds. (1988, April 29). *Science,* p. 579.

Jesser, C. J. (1978). Male responses to direct verbal sexual initiatives of females. *Journal of Sex Research, 14,* 118–128.

Kelly, J. A., St. Lawrence, J. S., Hood, H. V., & Brasfield, T. L. (1989). Behavioral intervention to reduce AIDS risk activities. *Journal of Consulting and Clinical Psychology, 57,* 60–67.

Komarovsky, M. (1976). *Dilemmas of masculinity: A study of college youth.* New York: Norton.

Kutner, N. G., & Brogan, D. (1974). An investigation of sex-related slang vocabulary and sex-role orientation among male and female university students. *Journal of Marriage and the Family, 36,* 474–484.

Larson, S. G. (1991). Television's mixed messages: Sexual content on "All My Children." *Communication Quarterly, 39,* 156–163.

Laws, J. L., & Schwartz, P. (1977). *Sexual scripts: The social construction of female sexuality.* Hinsdale, IL: The Dryden Press.

Maticka-Tyndale, E. (1991). Sexual scripts and AIDS prevention: Variations in adherence to safer-sex guidelines by heterosexual adolescents. *Journal of Sex Research, 28,* 45–66.

Mays, V. M., & Cochran, S. D. (1988). Issues in the perception of AIDS risk and risk reduction activities by Black and Hispanic/Latina women. *American Psychologist, 43,* 949–957.

McCormick, N. B. (1987). Sexual scripts: Social and therapeutic implications. *Sexual and Marital Therapy, 2,* 3–27.

McCormick, N. B., & Jesser, J. C. (1983). The courtship game: Power in the sexual encounter. In E. R. Allgeier & N. B. McCormick (Eds.), *Changing boundaries: Gender roles and sexual behavior* (pp. 64–86). Palo Alto, CA: Mayfield.

Metts, S., Cupach, W. R. (1991, May). *Plans for seeking and resisting the use of condoms.* Paper presented at the International Communication Association Convention, Chicago, IL.

Metts, S., Cupach, W. R., & Imahori, T. T. (1992). Perceptions of sexual compliance-resisting messages in three types of cross-sex relationships. *Western Journal of Speech Communication, 56,* 1–17.

O'Keefe, B. J. (1991). Message design logic and the management of multiple goals. In K. Tracy (Ed.), *Understanding face-to-face interaction: Issues linking goals and discourse* (pp. 131–150). Hillsdale, NJ: Lawrence Erlbaum Associates.

Perper, T., & Weis, D. L. (1987). Proceptive and rejective strategies of U.S. and Canadian college women. *Journal of Sex Research, 23,* 455–480.

Reiss, I. L., & Leik, R. K. (1989). Evaluating strategies to avoid AIDS: Number of partners versus use of condoms. *Journal of Sex Research, 4,* 411–433.

Sanders, J. S., & Robinson, W. L. (1979). Talking and not talking about sex: Male and female vocabularies. *Journal of Communication, 29,* 22–30.

Simon, W., & Gagnon, J. H. (1987). A sexual scripts approach. In J. H. Geer & W. O'Donohue (Eds.), *Theories of human sexuality* (pp. 363–383). New York: Plenum Press.

Snyder, M., & Campbell, B. (1980). Testing hypotheses about other people: The role of the hypothesis. *Personality and Social Psychology Bulletin, 6,* 421–426.

Sonnex, C., Hart, G. J., Williams, P., & Adler, M. W. (1989). Condom use by heterosexuals attending a department of GUM: Attitudes and behaviour in the light of HIV infection. *Genitourinary Medicine, 65,* 248–251.

Sprecher, S. (1990). The impact of the threat of AIDS on heterosexual dating relationships. *Journal of Psychology & Human Sexuality, 3*(2), 3–23.

Zimmerman, R. S. (1989). AIDS: Social causes, patterns, cures, and problems. In K. McKinney & S. Sprecher (Eds.), *Human sexuality: The societal and interpersonal context* (pp. 286–317). Norwood, NJ: Ablex.

CHAPTER TWO

Predicting the Use of Condoms: Past Behavior, Norms, and the Sexual Partner

Yoshihisa Kashima
La Trobe University, Australia

Cynthia Gallois
Malcolm McCamish
The University of Queensland, Australia

It has been recognized for a number of years now that, in the absence of a vaccine or cure for AIDS, efforts to contain the spread of the epidemic must be concentrated on bringing about widespread behavior change. Changing sexual practices, and particularly convincing people to use condoms every time they have intercourse, has become a central goal of AIDS prevention and education programs. Most programs have focused on bringing about individual behavior change. Sexual intercourse, however, is one of the most cooperative and social behaviors in our repertoire, and it crucially depends on communication between partners.

Unfortunately, the AIDS epidemic has appeared in a social context where many aspects of sex and sexuality, including talking about or studying sexual behavior, have taboos associated with them. Thus, we know relatively little about the factors influencing sexual decision making and sexual practice. As a result, AIDS education programs have often been designed and implemented without an adequate theoretical or research base, even though a large research effort is under way in most Western countries. The importance of adapting and extending existing theory to accommodate the cooperative nature of sexual behavior, along with the negotiation and emotional communication that this implies, has become increasingly apparent over the past several years.

This chapter discusses an Australian project aimed at examining sexual decision making among heterosexual and homosexual men and women. Our theoretical framework in the project has been the Theory of

Reasoned Action (Ajzen & Fishbein, 1980; Fishbein & Ajzen, 1975) and its more recent extension, the Theory of Planned Behavior (Ajzen, 1985, 1988). We have concentrated in particular on the social influence aspect of the theory, which is encapsulated as subjective norm in the original theory (see later). As is seen in later sections, our results suggest that this component is complex and multifaceted, and that the theory can be extended to take more account of normative factors. Our results also highlight the role of communication between sexual partners in negotiating the rules of sexual encounters and between peers in constructing norms for appropriate behavior and attitudes about communication.

AIDS IN AUSTRALIA

The course of the AIDS epidemic and responses to it in Australia have some unusual features that have probably influenced the spread of HIV infection in this country. First, Australia has a small population (approximately 17 million people), but a highly diverse one (there are over 80 immigrant ethnolinguistic groups in the country, as well as the native Aboriginal groups, where over 100 languages are represented). The AIDS epidemic in Australia has followed the pattern of most Western countries, affecting homosexual men and IV drug users first (the proportion of people in these groups may be slightly lower in Australia than in the United States; see Ross, 1988). As in other countries, HIV infection is now beginning to spread into the non-drug using heterosexual population. Some ethnic groups, particularly Aborigines, may be at special risk, as a result of their numbers, isolation, or sexual practices.

Although the first deaths from AIDS in Australia occurred in 1983, several years after the disease was noticed in the United States, the epidemic is well established now. This delay in onset may be part of the explanation for the response to the disease here. AIDS has been constructed by the Australian federal government mainly as a health problem, rather than as a sexual or moral one. Community-based AIDS councils had been set up in most states (largely by the gay communities) by 1985. In addition, the federal government began a campaign relatively early in the epidemic, which has been supplemented by most states. A national AIDS education program began in 1986. This campaign has included the installation of needle exchanges in major centers. In addition, special buses are used to distribute condoms and needles in an outreach program aimed at street kids and drug users. Such programs may in part explain the lower incidence to date of reported HIV infection among injecting drug users in Australia than in most other Western countries. There appears to have been less impact on sexual practices, however.

The first television ad produced by the federal government, aimed at raising awareness about AIDS and promoting the use of condoms, may go down as the most frightening such message anywhere in the world. The ad depicted AIDS as the medieval Grim Reaper, using bowling balls in a 10-pin alley to destroy men, women, children, and infants. Evaluations of this ad (Crawford, Kippax, & Tulloch, 1991; Ross, Rigby, Rosser, Brown, & Anagnostou, 1990) indicate that it did raise awareness and may have resulted in slightly more tolerant attitudes toward homosexuals and people with AIDS. It did not, however, produce behavior change in the direction of safer sex, although many people whose behavior was low risk asked for HIV-antibody testing. Since that time, television ads and written material have used lower levels of fear, but there is still a strong emphasis on the dangers of unsafe sex.

At the present time, AIDS is viewed by most people who have been surveyed in Australia as a very severe disease, perhaps the most severe of all (e.g., Heaven, 1987; Peterson & Peterson, 1987; Wright, 1990). In addition, knowledge about means of transmission and prevention is reasonable among many groups in the population, although knowledge of nontransmission is not as good (Crawford, Turtle, & Kippax, 1990; McCamish, Gallois, Arklay, & Wright, 1989; Rosenthal, Moore, & Brumen, 1990). As it is in many countries, however, AIDS seems to be perceived as a dread risk (Weinstein, 1989). This means that the perceived severity of the disease and knowledge about it do not predict preventive behavior.

Several studies indicate that a large proportion of gay men in Australia have made the change to safer sexual behavior (e.g., Connell et al., 1989; McCamish, Cox, Frazer, & North, 1988). Despite the increase in knowledge and awareness of HIV infection and AIDS, however, there has been little in the way of change to safer sexual practices among heterosexual students, the main heterosexual group studied. Indeed, one study (Turtle et al., 1989) found that students believed that they should engage in safer practices, and they knew what these practices were. Results for a matched group, however, indicated that the majority did not in fact use condoms for sex, even with casual partners. These results attest first to the importance for researchers of inquiring about actual behavior, rather than only beliefs or intentions. Second, there is a need for a more subtle understanding of the influences on sexual decisions, both where immediate short-term risk of infection is high and where it is lower.

HEALTH BELIEF MODELS

There are many possible causes for a reluctance to change behavior even when change is in the best interests of the person. Health belief models (e.g., Becker, Drachman, & Kirscht, 1974; Kirscht & Joseph, 1989; Rosenstock, 1974) have for many years pointed to the role of psychological variables, particularly the perception of risk or susceptibility, as crucial variables in the decision to adopt health-promoting behavior.

In the case of AIDS, many studies, including our own research, have shown that most people in all behavioral risk groups perceive themselves to be at low risk of infection (see Weinstein, 1989, for a review of research on optimistic bias as a general phenomenon). Some factors reduce this feeling of confidence that one is at low risk of infection. Members of groups where the prevalence of HIV infection is higher are aware that they are at somewhat higher risk. In our studies, for example, homosexual men typically perceived themselves to be at higher risk of HIV infection than did heterosexuals (Gallois, Timmins, McCamish, Terry, & Kashima, 1991). Personal contact with someone who has HIV or AIDS also personalizes the sense of risk. We found that personal contact with people with HIV resulted in higher ratings of personal risk for both heterosexual and homosexual men. Nevertheless, all groups of participants in our studies rated their risk as much lower than average, and as lower than for their same-sex or their opposite-sex friends.

Recent versions of health belief models have stressed the influence of factors other than risk assessment. Self-efficacy (see Bandura, 1989, for a discussion of self-efficacy in the context of AIDS prevention) and the acquisition of skills necessary for safer sex (Fisher & Fisher, 1990) have been included, as has a calculation of the benefits of safer sex and the barriers to it (Bauman & Siegel, 1987, review these barriers for homosexual men; Siegel & Gibson, 1988, present a similar analysis for heterosexuals). The Morin model (Morin & Batchelor, 1984; Puckett & Bye, 1987), which has been the most widely used theoretical basis for AIDS-prevention programs in gay communities, adds two other important variables: the perception that safer sex is satisfying, and the belief that one has the support of peers in adopting safer practices. Fisher (1988) also discussed the informational and normative role of peers in AIDS prevention.

THEORY OF REASONED ACTION
AND RECENT EXTENSIONS

The Theory of Reasoned Action (Ajzen & Fishbein, 1980; Fishbein & Ajzen, 1975) incorporates most of the variables included in health belief models into a predictive theory of behavior change. Fishbein and Ajzen argued that the most important direct influence on the enactment of any behavior is the intention to engage in the behavior, especially if the measurement of intention and behavior are very close in time. Intention in its turn is predicted by a person's attitude toward the behavior. Attitude is a summary of the perceived costs and benefits (often called *evaluations*) of enacting the behavior and is predicted by the sum of these costs and benefits, each multiplied by its perceived likelihood of occurrence. Intention is also predicted by the subjective norm with regard to the behavior, which is a summary statement of what the actor believes important other people think he or she should do. Subjective norm is predicted by the sum of these normative beliefs for each significant other person, multiplied by the actor's motivation to comply with that person. In the original version of the theory, these were proposed to be the only salient influences on the adoption or not of a new behavior. The theory has received a good deal of empirical support, for example in predicting cessation of smoking (Budd, 1986), alcohol consumption (Kilty, 1978), contraceptive use (Davidson & Jaccard, 1979), the use of condoms (Fisher, 1984; Middlestadt & Fishbein, 1990), and safer sex among gay men (Ross & McLaws, in press).

In a recent application of the Theory of Reasoned Action to AIDS-preventive behavior, Fishbein and Middlestadt (1989) again pointed to the specific and local nature of the variables in the theory. First, different groups of people may perceive the same behavior to have different costs and benefits, and they may be influenced by different people. In the case of sex, experienced and inexperienced people differ in the central importance of the sexual partner. In addition, for some groups, the behavior may be more under the influence of norms, whereas for others, it may be more under attitudinal control. For example, McLaws, Ross, Oldenberg, and Cooper (1989) found that for gay men, the relative importance of attitudes and norms in predicting intentions about safer sex varied as a function of age. Similarly, Middlestadt and Fishbein (1990) found that the intention to use a condom was predicted mainly by normative factors for sexually experienced women, but by attitudes for inexperienced women.

The situation also changes as a function of the type of behavior. Smoking or weight loss, for example, involve mainly behavior by only one person, although the person may be influenced by others. Sexual behaviors are more cooperative, and generally require action (or at least permission to act) by both partners. In the case of condom use, cooperation must often be negotiated. Sexual partners, therefore, must perceive that they are free, and that they have the skills, to discuss their feelings and worries with each other when this is necessary (Fisher & Fisher, 1990). To maintain safer behavior, they must also find a way to incorporate it that does not detract from their sexual communication or the satisfaction they receive from sex. For example, Gold, Skinner, Grant, and Plummer (in press), in an Australian study of gay men, found that a factor that significantly differentiated between unsafe sexual encounters and encounters where the respondent had been tempted to have unsafe sex but had actually had safer sex was the amount of communication about safer sex between the partners. In this study, communication involved direct discussion, indirect discussion, or nonverbal signals. The important thing was that it occurred.

The Theory of Reasoned Action implies that intervention programs aiming to bring about health-promoting behavior need to take at least the following factors into account: the specific group of people at which interventions are targeted, the type of behavior that is targeted for change, and the causal influences on the intentions relevant to this behavior. The theory provides a conceptual and methodological framework within which interventions can be designed and evaluated. Figure 2.1 presents the major components of the theory.

Nonetheless, there are some limitations to the theory as it presently stands. First, the scope of the theory is by design limited to behaviors that are largely under volitional control (Ajzen has dealt with this issue to some extent by involving the concept of behavioral control; see later). Second, the theory postulates only one normative factor, subjective norm, that influences intentions along with attitudes. The previous discussion suggests that there are more normative influences than this. Third, the theory is cast within a framework of individual decision making, even though many social behaviors require a high degree of communication and cooperation between people. In the case of sexual behavior, the role of the interaction with sexual partner must be examined very carefully.

Theory of Planned Behavior: Predicting Goal-Directed Behavior

Social behavior is not always controlled by the intentions of individual actors. Sometimes, we cannot do what we intend. Ajzen and his colleagues (Ajzen, 1985, 1988; Ajzen & Madden, 1986; Schifter & Ajzen, 1985) have expanded the Theory of Reasoned Action to what they call the Theory of Planned Behavior, with a view to predicting a greater range of behavior. According to these researchers, most social acts are not under complete volitional control, but should be conceptualized as a composite of behaviors and goals. For instance, losing weight can be called a behavior-goal unit, which consists of both a variety of behaviors (such as exercising and dieting) and the goal of weight reduction. In order to lose weight, one must exercise and diet. Whether these behaviors enable one to attain the goal of weight reduction depends on many things, such as adequate physiological processes. Ajzen (1988) summarized these external

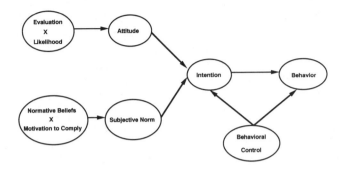

FIG. 2.1.   Relationships between attitudes, norms, intention, and behavior, as predicted by the Theory of Reasoned Action/Theory of Planned Behavior (after Ajzen, 1985; Fishbein & Ajzen, 1975).

factors under the rubrics of opportunity and dependence on other people. Some of them involve other behaviors by the actor (e.g., learning about an effective diet), but some events are outside the control of the actor.

Ajzen (1985; Ajzen & Madden, 1986) called *behavioral control* the extent to which an actor can control intervening events, as well as the extent to which the antecedent conditions necessary for performing the behavior are satisfied. When there are few intervening events between behavior and goal attainment, the amount of control an actor has over a behavior is largely reduced to the satisfaction of *behavioral conditions.* For example, the fact that someone has a condom available and an agreement with his or her sexual partner to use condoms for intercourse means that the person is in a position to use a condom. Once a condom is worn, the goal is attained. Thus, behavioral control in this case is reduced to the extent to which behavioral conditions are satisfied.

In addition, Ajzen and his colleagues have suggested that the intention to perform a behavior predicts the actor's attempts at performing the behavior. Thus, because of the lack of behavioral control, intention may not predict goal attainment. But, given the intention, the actor is likely to start performing a series of behaviors that may lead to the goal. For example, the intention to use a condom is likely to be a good predictor of satisfying the behavioral conditions of obtaining a condom and negotiating an agreement with the sexual partner to use one.

Role of Past Behavior

A number of studies (Bentler & Speckart, 1979, 1981; Fredericks & Dossett, 1983; Manstead, Proffitt, & Smart, 1983) have shown that another variable, past behavior, appears to have an independent influence on behavior, and this influence is not completely mediated by intention. These findings suggest that past behavior is an important element in behavioral control, and may be an influence in the satisfaction of behavioral conditions. In addition, past behavior may interact with intention in determining actual behavior; that is, whether men and women have used condoms for sex in the past may predict their having condoms available, their making an agreement with their sexual partners to use condoms, and this variable may also interact with their intention to use a condom the next time they have intercourse. There are a number of reasons for this interaction.

Past behavior is, we believe, a strong stabilizer of intentions. When a person performs a behavior, the person makes a commitment, and commitment is likely to decrease the likelihood of changing one's mind. In addition, people who have performed a behavior before are likely to have a greater amount of information about the performance of the behavior. Intentions supported with more information should be more stable, and new contradictory information is likely to have a smaller effect (Anderson, 1967; Davidson, Yantis, Norwood, & Montano, 1985; Wood, 1982). Finally, a person who has already performed a behavior has directly experienced the behavior, rather than simply thinking about it. As Fazio and his colleagues (Fazio, Powell, & Herr, 1983; Fazio & Zanna, 1981) have shown, attitudes formed on the basis of direct experience are likely to have properties that are markedly different from attitudes formed without direct experience. One of these properties is stability (Wu & Shaffer, 1987).

In addition to its stabilizing effect on intention, past behavior influences the extent to which behavioral conditions are satisfied. As we noted earlier, the satisfaction of behavioral conditions is a part of the behavioral control described by the Theory of Planned Behavior. The satisfaction of behavioral conditions operates as a threshold. When behavioral conditions are not satisfied, the behavior cannot be performed. For example, if a condom is not available when a couple has sex, they cannot use a condom. Thus, they are forced to change intentions (Fishbein & Ajzen, 1975). On the other hand, if someone has performed a given behavior at least once before, he or she must have satisfied the necessary behavioral conditions. In this case, the person must have decided to use a condom, bought one, and had it available. Past behavior, then, is likely to be a good indicator of whether a person is able to satisfy the behavioral conditions again for a performance of the same behavior in future.

NORMS AND THE THEORY OF REASONED ACTION

As we noted earlier, subjective norms are not the only normative factor that influences intentions. Researchers such as Schwartz and Tessler (1972), Kilty (1978), Pagel and Davidson (1984), Budd and Spencer (1985), and Kashima and Kashima (1988) argue that *personal norms* should also be included. Personal norms involve the actor's own sense of normative pressure (i.e., I think I should perform the behavior), rather than the pressure of significant others' opinions. Ajzen and Fishbein (1973) thought that personal norms were empirically indistinguishable from intention. Other researchers have found that they are distinguishable. Budd and Spencer recently suggested that personal norms can be viewed as ideal behavioral intentions: what the actor would do under ideal circumstances.

In addition, Grube, Morgan, and McGree (1986) suggested that *behavioral norms* should be included in the prediction of intentions. Behavioral norms are actors' perceptions about whether significant others perform the behavior themselves. Many researchers in the area of behavior change have found that people's decisions are strongly influenced by whether their friends and peers are perceived to do the same thing. In the area of AIDS-preventive behavior, Fisher (1988) described social networks as having safer or unsafe norms. In his view, these norms consist to a large extent of perceptions and communication about the behavior of peers. Behavioral norms are conceptually different from subjective norms, in that the former have to do with what significant others are perceived to do, whereas the latter are presumably concerned with what others say the actor should do. Again, the concept of behavioral norms highlights communication, this time between friends and peers.

Researchers have also suggested that the Theory of Reasoned Action does not take sufficient account of the interactive effects of attitudinal and normative factors on intentions. Andrews and Kandel (1979), Liska (1984), Bagozzi and Schnedlitz (1985), and Grube et al. (1986) have pointed out that people's intentions to perform a behavior are enhanced when their attitude is positive toward the behavior and social norms are supportive of the performance of the behavior. Intentions to perform the behavior are weakened when this is not the case. In short, attitudes and social norms are proposed to have an interactive effect on intentions.

ROLE OF THE SEXUAL PARTNER

As Liska (1984) noted and Fishbein and Ajzen (1975) recognized, the performance of social behaviors often requires cooperation. The partner in a cooperative behavior potentially plays three distinct roles in decision making. First, the partner may act as an influence on the attitude toward the behavior. If an actor expects that a behavior may cause some unpleasantness in the partner or the partner may not like it, the actor's attitude to performing the behavior is likely to be more negative. This suggests that the partner's wish influences intentions indirectly through attitudes. Second, the partner may be seen as one of the very important persons in the actor's social environment who can provide reward or punishment. Thus, the partner's wish may influence intentions indirectly through norms, especially the subjective norm. Third, the partner's cooperation may be seen as a necessary condition for the performance of cooperative behavior. The actor's belief as to whether the partner thinks he or she should or should not perform the behavior can be conceptualized as one of the social constraints on the behavior, a part of behavioral control. Severe social constraints mean that the actor is forced to change intentions, regardless of his or her attitudes and norms about the behavior (Ajzen, 1985, 1988). Unless such social constraints are extremely enduring and initiate changes in attitudes and norms, beliefs about them may influence intentions directly, independently of attitudes and norms.

At this juncture, Budd and Spencer's suggestion that personal norms should be seen as ideal intentions sheds new light on the conceptualization of the partner's wish. An intention to use a condom for intercourse may be strong if the ideal intention (personal norm about condom use) is strong and the person believes that his or her sexual partner has the same beliefs. This suggests that intentions may be mainly a function of what the actor would ideally do and what the actor believes the partner wants to do.

A STUDY OF CONDOM USE IN AUSTRALIA

The project presented in this chapter involves an examination of social factors that influence decisions about using a condom. We have examined an extension of the Theory of Reasoned Action/Theory of Planned Behavior, which is presented later in Fig. 2.2. We review some of the major results from the project, which are reported in more detail elsewhere. Specifically, we examine the impact of past condom use on intentions and behavior, as well as the effects of different types of norms, the interactive effects of attitudes and norms on intentions, and the role of the sexual partner. Our results and others like them, we believe, have important implications for AIDS education programs and, in particular, for the communication skills that form a part of such programs. In addition, our results lead to an expansion of several components in the Theory of Reasoned Action.

Pilot Study

A central premise of the Theory of Reasoned Action is that groups of people differ not only in their intentions toward a particular behavior, but also in the costs and benefits they associate with the behavior and the others who influence their thinking about the behavior. Therefore, it is important to determine the evaluations and significant others that are salient to participants before attempting either to study or to change behavior. This exercise seems especially important in the case of sexual behavior, given the taboos that exist in most Western societies about talking about sex and the general lack of scientific knowledge about sexual practices.

For this project, we conducted a pilot study with 24 homosexual and heterosexual men (mean age = 27.8 years) and women (mean age = 24.8 years). These volunteers were selected to be similar in age and social class to participants in the main studies. They took part in semi-structured interviews, where they were asked to describe their own sexual practices and other practices they knew about. They indicated what they thought were the most important advantages and disadvantages for each practice. In addition, they named other people who were important to their decisions about sexual matters, and indicated whether they were inclined to do what these people wanted them to (thus establishing whether the influence was positive or negative). Finally, they indicated activities associated with sex that they felt would increase or decrease the chances of contracting HIV or another sexually transmitted disease (STD). From these interviews, we obtained a list of 6 sexual practices that were important to several of the pilot subjects, 13 associated costs and benefits, 6 significant others, and 12 related activities. These were included in the main questionnaires described later.

Main Studies

We conducted two parallel studies. The first made use of a sample drawn from the general community in Brisbane; the second was conducted with young undergraduates. All participants in both studies were currently sexually active. The studies were prospective in design. Questions concerning attitudes and norms, intentions, and past behavior were assessed at one session, and questions about behavior were answered after each participant's next sexual encounter and returned to us by post.

Participants and Procedure. Participants in the first study were 85 heterosexual men (mean age = 27.4 years), 85 heterosexual women (mean age = 26.7 years), and 82 homosexual men (mean age = 31.2 years), who volunteered to participate. These people were matched in age and occupation from people in a larger sample who completed both parts of the study. Lesbians and bisexuals were not included in this study because they numbered fewer than 30 per group. Participants were recruited through social organizations (particularly organizations for gay men) and through subjects' social networks. Most of the participants were native to Queensland, and three quarters of them lived in Brisbane, a city of about 1 million people and the state capital. Three quarters of the survey participants said they were Christians, but they were not very religious. The majority of participants in all three groups had at least some tertiary education and were employed in professional or clerical jobs, so that they should be thought of as middle class.

In the second study, we selected a sample of young male and female university students. These people were specifically targeted because they have a special need for education in safer sexual behavior. One hundred forty sexually active undergraduate students (71 males and 69 females), aged between 17 and 21 years (mean age = 18.1 years), volunteered to participate in the study for course credit and completed both questionnaires. All subjects in this study described themselves as exclusively heterosexual in orientation.

Participants completed the initial questionnaire as part of a large-scale survey about sexual behavior. This questionnaire asked for demographic information and a history of sexual behavior, as well as present and intended sexual practices and attitudes about various aspects of sexual behavior and safer sex. It was completed in a face-to-face session with the interviewer; subjects were either alone or in a small group. Participants were given a follow-up questionnaire to return after their next sexual encounter. This questionnaire inquired about their actual sexual behavior on that occasion. If they had not had a sexual contact within 4 weeks, they returned the follow-up questionnaire blank (these people were eliminated from the statistical analyses).

Measures.   As we noted earlier, the questionnaires enquired about participants' present sexual practices, as well as their intentions, beliefs, attitudes, and norms about various sexual activities that may increase or reduce risk of contracting STDs (e.g., sex in an exclusive relationship, sex with a new partner, consuming alcohol or other drugs during sex). The two studies used questionnaires that were similar in design, but that had some differences in specific questions.

In both studies, intention to use a condom was measured by items asking subjects whether they intended for themselves or their sexual partner to wear a condom the next time they had sex. Past behavior with regard to condom use was examined by asking subjects to indicate the percentage of their past sexual contacts in which they or their partner wore a condom. Participants also indicated whether they had used a condom the last time they had sex. In addition, two items on the first questionnaire and another two items on the follow-up questionnaire were used to index the extent to which the behavioral conditions necessary for condom use were satisfied. These items asked whether subjects had obtained a condom so that it would be available for their sexual contact, and whether they had made an agreement with their sexual partner to use a condom. Participants were also asked whether they were in a sexually exclusive relationship and for the number of their sexual partners in the past year (exclusivity was defined by us as no more than one partner in the past year). Actual behavior was measured on the follow-up questionnaire by a dichotomous item asking whether the subject or partner had worn a condom.

In the second study, participants' attitudes toward using a condom the next time they had sex were measured by asking whether sex with a condom was unpleasant–pleasant and dull–exciting. Subjective norm was measured with an item asking about the degree to which "People who are important to me think I should perform my sexual activities with me or my partner wearing a condom." The items measuring personal norm asked whether participants personally thought they or their partners should use a condom the next time they had sex. Participants were also asked to report how many friends of theirs they thought would use a condom (behavioral norms).

Sexual Practices Relevant to Condom Use.   The heterosexuals in the study almost all had vaginal intercourse, with very few having anal intercourse. These numbers are not surprising for a sexually active group of heterosexuals, except that the number of people having anal sex is lower than the often-quoted figure of 10%. Turtle et al. (1989) and Crawford et al. (1990), in studies of Australian students in their 20s, found about 7% of their subjects reporting anal intercourse, mainly in regular relationships. These results may indicate a trend away from this practice among Australian middle-class heterosexuals. For homosexual men, only a minority of participants were having anal sex, which supports findings from other Australian studies that show a drop in the popularity of anal sex among gay men (e.g., Connell et al., 1989; McCamish et al., 1988). Connell et al. found a strong link between desire for anal sex and age, with the popularity of this practice being very low among young men. Such a change in the popularity of anal sex has still-unexplored implications for the negotiation of safer sex among gay men, especially where there is an age difference between partners.

Only minorities of each group of participants used condoms, either in the past or on the occasion studied. For homosexual men, this did not affect the safety of their sexual practice, as the vast majority of men having anal sex (about 90%) did use condoms. For heterosexuals, however, about 45% of our participants were relying on exclusive relationships to protect themselves, and 30% of men and women took no precautions at all (see Gallois, Kashima, Hills, & McCamish, 1990; Gallois et al., in press, for more details). This is a somewhat worrying situation, given that exclusivity for young unmarried heterosexuals (over 75% of our heterosexual participants were single) tends to mean serial monogamy, often of no more than several months duration (see Rosenthal et al., 1990).

PREDICTING BEHAVIOR:
PAST BEHAVIOR AND INTENTIONS

In order to assess the contribution of past behavior and intentions in predicting behavior, a hierarchical multiple regression analysis was conducted for the total sample in Study 1, with actual behavior as the criterion variable, intention and past behavior as predictors in the first step, and their product as a predictor in the second step (see Kashima, Gallois, Hills, & McCamish, 1991, for more details). Both intention and past behavior were significant predictors, and their interaction significantly increased prediction in the second step. Next, the interactive effect of intention and past behavior was examined separately for each group in the sample. For both the heterosexual men and women, the main and interaction effects were significant. For the homosexual men, the results were in the same direction, but only past behavior was a significant predictor. These results were replicated for participants in Study 2. Essentially, the interactions indicated that if participants had used condoms in the past and they intended to do so the next time, they were more likely to use a condom the next time they had sex. If they did not intend to use a condom, they were unlikely to do so. Those who had not used condoms in the past, however, were unlikely to do so the next time, whether they intended to use a condom or not.

The story was more complex than it appeared at first, however. To explore further the way in which past behavior and intention combined to produce condom use or non-use, we divided those participants in Study 1 who indicated that they intended to practice anal or vaginal sex into two groups: those who intended to use condoms and those who did not (Gallois et al., in press). We found that for nonintenders, past behavior seemed to stabilize intention. If past behavior and intentions were similar (those who had not used condoms in the past and did not intend to do so), the intention was much more likely to be carried out than when past behavior and intentions were different. Condom intenders, on the other hand, were not as stable. Whether they had used condoms in the past or not, only about half of them carried out their intention to do so. Clearly, some factor was preventing these people from practicing safer sex. Further analyses were conducted to explore the role of attitudes and norms, as well as the satisfaction of behavioral conditions, in this relationship. Then, we focused on the role of the sexual partner.

Behavioral Conditions for Condom Use

According to our theoretical analysis, the satisfaction of necessary behavioral conditions acts as a threshold function. When behavioral conditions are satisfied beyond a certain level, the behavior may occur; otherwise, the behavior is unlikely to occur. To test this prediction, we looked at participants in Study 2, who had answered more detailed questions about condom use (see Kashima, Gallois, Hills, & McCamish, 1991, for more details). The proportion of respondents who used a condom was computed for each of four levels of satisfaction of the conditions: (a) neither of the conditions (having a condom available and making an agreement with the sexual partner to use one) was satisfied, (b) no condom was available but an agreement was made, (c) a condom was available but no agreement was made, and (d) a condom was available and an agreement was made.

The proportion of condom users increased as the level of satisfying the necessary conditions increased. At the first level, none of the 55 subjects used a condom, and at the second level, none of the 12 used a condom. At the third level, 30.8% (4 out of 13) used a condom, and at the fourth level, 70.9% (39 out of 55) did so. This implies that the availability of a condom was an absolutely necessary condition for condom use. The second condition, having an agreement with the partner to use a condom, also greatly increased the probability of condom use, but it was not an absolutely necessary condition. Therefore, we recoded the responses for subsequent analyses: those who did not have a condom = 1, those who had a condom but not an agreement = 2, and those who had both a condom and an agreement = 3.

Intention, condition, and the product of these after centering were entered to a multiple regression to predict actual behavior. As expected, the model was significant and all predictors had significant beta weights. Thus, satisfaction of behavioral conditions also interacted with intention in predicting behavior. In addition, past behavior and intention were both significant predictors of the extent to which the behavioral conditions were satisfied. Thus, people who had used condoms in the past, and who intended to do so again, were very likely to have a condom available and an agreement with their partner.

Finally, the stabilizing effect of past behavior on intention was tested separately for each level of satisfaction of behavioral conditions, by examining the interactive effect of intention and past behavior on actual behavior. At the first level, in which a condom was not available, none of the subjects used a condom. At the second level, results were not significant, because of the small sample size. At the third level, in which a condom was available and an agreement was made, past behavior, intention, and their product were significant predictors of behavior.

ATTITUDES, NORMS, AND THE SEXUAL PARTNER

For participants in both studies, the sexual partner was far and away the most important person influencing decisions about sex (Gallois et al., 1990). Next came friends and peers, who were still a considerable influence. Well behind these two types of people were parents, siblings, and the general public. In addition, participants believed their sexual partners approved of their sexual practices more than other people did. Interestingly, heterosexual men were less sure of the approval of their partner than were women. Males were also more worried about doing something their female partners may not like. Finally, the perception of the sexual partner's norm was significantly correlated with the participant's attitude toward using a condom, as well as with subjective norm.

Some specific differences suggested that condom users may be more worried about their practices than non-users. First, condom users (as well as those who practiced nonpenetrative sex) felt that they had less approval from their parents and siblings for what they were doing. They also felt they would be less intimate with their partners than non-users. Condom users who were not in exclusive relationships, however, were less worried about causing pain and discomfort to their partners than were other participants. All of this suggests that condom users may be less sure of the normative support they have, and more dependent on their partners for support.

Predicting Intentions

As noted earlier, the Theory of Reasoned Action proposes that intentions are predicted by the actor's attitude and subjective norm toward the behavior. In addition, we were interested in the effect on intentions of personal norms, behavioral norms, and most particularly the partner's norm. We examined the effects of these variables, and the interaction of the other variables with personal norm, via a hierarchical multiple regression analysis for participants in Study 2 (see Kashima, Gallois, & McCamish, 1991, for more details). We suspected that there may be a sex difference, as a man wears a condom, and his refusal would constrain the use of a condom more strongly than his partner's wish. Many writers have also commented on the power difference in sexual relationships, and its impact on sexual decision making.

For men, personal norms and the interaction of attitude and behavioral norms were significant psychological contributors to intention. Men's intentions to use a condom were enhanced if they thought they should use one and if their attitude was backed up by their observation that their friends and peers also used condoms. For women, on the other hand, partner norms, personal norms, and the interaction between these two were significant predictors. This implies that women intend to have their partner wear a condom if they think they should use a condom and if their partner is seen to be willing. Although the sex difference in these results was small, it does indicate that the men in the study were paying relatively more attention to what they believed their friends were doing, whereas the women were relatively more attentive to their partner's perceived wishes.

Even though men may be very concerned about their partner and about doing something she may not like (indeed, more concerned than women are), they may gather information about what to do more from other sources than the partner. Other researchers have also found that men are very concerned about their partner's wishes and satisfaction, but that they may not talk very much about these (Waldby, Kippax, & Crawford, 1990). In addition, Waldby et al. concluded that men seem to gather information about sex to a greater extent from books and other external sources than do women. Overall, these results suggest a lack of communication between heterosexual partners about the use of condoms, which may undermine the intention to use them. This conclusion is supported by Fisher's (1990) study of heterosexual young people. Fisher found that both men and women expressed a wish to use condoms, but did not do so because they feared their partner would not want to.

Finally, past behavior was added to see whether it improved the prediction of intentions. For men, the percentage of variance accounted for significantly increased, but the addition of past behavior did not change the pattern of results. For women, the effect of past behavior was completely mediated by the intervening variables. Two possible reasons for this sex difference are offered here. First, the direct link of past behavior to intention for men may be eliminated if other intervening variables are identified; the effect of past behaviors for women was effectively eliminated with the identification of the interaction between partner norm and personal norm. Second, it is possible that men's decisions to use condoms may be made more mindlessly than women's. Men may tend to intend to do what they did in the past, whereas women may think more about this decision.

IMPLICATIONS FOR THEORY AND RESEARCH

The results of our research and other studies show the usefulness of the
Theory of Reasoned Action in understanding and predicting sexual decision making. As we noted earlier, this theory incorporates many of the
variables that appear in most versions of the health-belief model. The Theory of Reasoned Action also places more emphasis on the role of attitudes and social influence in decisions about behavior. Nonetheless, the
theory can usefully be expanded to a more general framework, to capture the full complexity of social behavior.

Our results suggest that the social (normative) component should be
expanded in several ways. It is worth pointing out that not many studies
have explored the way that social influences affect this model. Like attitudes, norms are complex variables that influence different behaviors in
different ways. We examined three types of norms: subjective, personal,
and behavioral. These norms appear to have different consequences, and
to represent different aspects of normative pressure. Different types of
norms are also predicted in different ways. Subjective norm is predicted
by beliefs about what others think we should do (Fishbein & Ajzen, 1975);
behavioral norms, by our perceptions about what our peers do; and personal norms, by a combination of attitudes and subjective norms (Kashima, Gallois, & McCamish, 1991). Figure 2.2 sketches some of the
relationships our results point to.

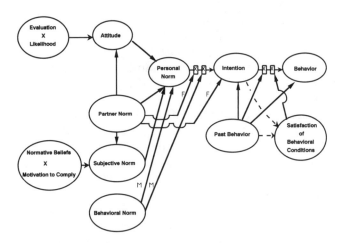

FIG. 2.2.   Relationships between variables found in our results and predicted by our extension of the Theory of Reasoned Action/Theory of Planned
Behavior (X = interaction between variables; M = found for men only;
F = found for women only; solid lines indicate relationships established
empirically; dashed lines indicate predicted relationships).

Overall, subjective, personal, and behavioral norms can be differentiated according to two facets. First, subjective and behavioral norms pertain to the actor's perceptions of others, whereas personal norms have to do with the actor's own sense of normative obligation. Second, subjective and personal norms have to do with thoughts and beliefs, whereas behavioral norms are concerned with behavior, as their name implies. When the various types of norms are combined, a two by two classification of norms is formed:

	Perspective	
	Self	Other(s)
Thinking	Personal norm	Subjective norm
Doing	——	Behavioral norm

The missing quadrant, where the actor's behavior provides some impetus to intentions or behavior, is not ordinarily called a norm. What seems to fit best here is the actor's past behavior.

It is likely that different strategies are necessary to change these different norms. For example, behavioral norms may change as a result of communication from friends, especially opinion leaders. Kelly, St. Lawrence, and their colleagues (Kelly et al., 1990) described an innovative program in which opinion leaders were identified in gay communities. These people were trained to communicate safer-sex messages, which included messages about their personal behavior. Kelly et al.'s results showed that the introduction of trained opinion leaders led to safer sexual behavior among the whole population of gay men in the community. This may have been largely due to a change in behavioral norms brought about by the opinion leaders. Such a strategy may also lead to a change in personal norms if attitude change is involved. It is less likely to have an impact on subjective norms, however. In this case, direct communication about the person's own behavior, particularly by the sexual partner, may be necessary. At this stage, these are hypotheses that must be examined by future research. The study of norms about sexual practice and the ways in which they are communicated is a fruitful area for research within this theoretical tradition.

Our results add some complexity to the causal paths specified in the Theory of Reasoned Action (see Fig. 2.2), some of which have already been suggested by the Theory of Planned Behavior. It is already well known that intentions do not always predict behavior, and many questions can be raised about the intention–behavior link. An examination of necessary conditions for carrying out an intention, and an understanding of the events that intervene between behavior and goal attainment, are both crucial to extending the conceptualization of the intention–behavior relationship.

The role of past behavior, in particular, appears to be central to understanding sexual practice in general, and the use of condoms in particular. Our studies show that past behavior stabilizes the intention to use a condom (or to practice another form of safer sex, such as nonpenetrative sex). In addition, past behavior predicts the satisfaction of two conditions necessary for condom use: having a condom available and making an agreement with one's partner to use it. There may be other such necessary conditions, of course, for other populations. For example, Ross and McLaws (in press) found that assertive skills interacted with intention in the prediction of safer sexual practice in a sample of gay men. Clearly, communication skills are necessary for negotiating any agreement with the sexual partner, given that even the discussion of sex in private is filled with taboos. In any case, further refinement of the concept of behavioral conditions is another task for future researchers in this area.

Once again, we point to the importance of determining the influences on specific behaviors for specific groups of people. As Fishbein and Middlestadt (1987, 1989) proposed, people differ both in the content of their attitudes and norms about a behavior and in the relative influence of these variables. Our results indicate that the sexual practices of younger and older sexually active people may not be influenced to the same extent by norms and attitudes. In addition, neither attitudes nor norms correlated very well with intentions about safer sex for the gay men in our sample. Instead, past behavior was a central influence. It may be that these men, who in general practiced safer sex of one sort or another, did so no matter how they felt about it, as a reaction to the short-term risk of unsafe behavior.

As Fishbein and Middlestadt (1989) pointed out, it is essential to determine the specific beliefs that underpin attitudes, the significant others that underpin norms, and the most salient behavior for particular groups, before designing intervention programs to promote safer sex. The pilot study we conducted, which gathered qualitative data about the groups we were studying, is an essential phase of research using the Theory of Reasoned Action, as well as an essential part of educational interventions. Researchers and educators must understand the salient features of the people they work with; otherwise, the research or the interventions are likely to fail.

Finally, the causal relationships postulated by the Theory of Reasoned Action and the Theory of Planned Behavior must be checked. At present, it is necessary to assume that the basic premises of the theory are correct in order to design a study or an intervention based on them. A task for future researchers is to conduct experimental tests of the basic propositions, either in the laboratory or in the field. Such experiments should include examination of the communication processes implicated by our results.

SOCIALIZING THE USE OF CONDOMS

Our results point to the importance of satisfying behavioral conditions for the practice of safer sex. Some help in this direction can come from the larger society. For example, in order to use a condom, one needs to have one. Various strategies can be used to make condoms more available, such as the installation of condom vending machines (so that people do not have to communicate with pharmacists), free distribution of condoms by various agencies, and so forth. Before carrying out such interventions, however, a detailed study of the behavioral conditions that are important for a specific group is desirable. For some groups, the availability of condoms and knowledge about how to use them may be more important than is negotiating an agreement with sexual partners to use them. For other groups, the opposite may be true.

Our results, taken together with the results of other research, indicate that social norms among young sexually active heterosexuals still do not favor the use of condoms as a way of reducing the risk of HIV transmission. Instead, those participants in our project who either relied on exclusivity or simply relied on chance to protect them felt that they had more support from others than did people who used condoms (Gallois et al., in press). This may also have been true to some extent even for the homosexual men in our study, who seemed to practice safer sex in spite of their attitudes, and who paid little attention to the norms of the larger community. Condom users may still be in the avant-garde, ahead of the community in which they live.

In the past year (since our data were collected), the Australian federal government has begun a mass media campaign aimed at socializing the use of condoms. One recent television ad depicts a couple in bed, with one partner reminding the other of their agreement to use condoms and sending the recalcitrant partner out to buy one. Another ad uses a *vox populi* format to show young men and women talking (favorably) about condoms in public. This approach would appear to be a helpful step in promoting the idea that using condoms is normal behavior.

Although mass media efforts may have some impact, most research shows clearly that behavior change is influenced more strongly, as the Theory of Reasoned Action proposes, by interpersonal factors. It is our friends and especially our sexual partners who shape our ideas about the pleasantness of condoms and about their usefulness. Our results indicate that these two types of people influence our personal norms about condoms and interact with them in influencing our intentions to use condoms. Normative change may begin at the mass level, but it actually takes place at the level of interpersonal communication.

A necessary condition for studying the impact of the peer group on norms, or for designing interventions to change norms through the peer group, involves determining who is in the peer group. This may have been done in the case of homosexual men, at least for those who are strongly identified with the gay community (Connell & Kippax, 1990; Puckett & Bye, 1987). It is still not really clear, however, who the peer group is for heterosexuals when they think or talk about sex. Our results indicate that the sexual partner is a crucial peer (perhaps especially for women), and that friends are the next most important group (especially for men; much less important than the partner, however). Future research is needed to elucidate this important domain.

CONCLUSION: TALKING ABOUT SEX

If social change at the interpersonal level is a more potent vehicle for behavioral change than change driven by mass appeals, then talking about sex may be the most important behavior in promoting safer sexual practice. A number of studies indicate that young people feel they can talk freely about sex, at least with their sexual partner, and that they will not do something they do not want to. For example, Abbott (1987) found that the large majority of adolescent women in her sample felt that they could speak freely about sex, and that they could refuse any activity they did not want to participate in, including unsafe sex. Crawford et al. (1990) and Wilders and MacCallum (1990) found similar results with older groups of men and women. Other studies, however, show that in fact people do not talk about their sexual norms, desires, or preferences (Fisher, 1990).

The taboos about sexual communication, thus, may affect practice more than they affect perceptions. This is an unfortunate state of affairs, as safer sex in general involves normative change. In addition, the necessary conditions we found for condom use involve communication about sex. To have a condom available, one must learn about condoms and must buy them from someone else. To make an agreement to use condoms, one must negotiate with the sexual partner.

As Fisher and Fisher (1990) pointed out, and as our results indicate, norms are more resistant to change if actors feel that significant others are continuing to follow older norms. Actors are unlikely to change their minds about this if they never talk about sexual norms. In addition, it is difficult for a person (particularly a woman) to assert her right to safer sex if she does not perceive a normative climate that favors safer sex. Most research on the effectiveness of assertive messages indicates that these messages are not likely to succeed if they are rule-violating. Thus, it is much easier to initiate a request for the use of condoms that is supported by norms than it is to refuse a request for unsafe sex that peers support.

In conclusion, our results point to the importance of social influences and communication on decisions, intentions, and behavior relevant to safer sex. Some research and intervention programs are aimed specifically at increasing communication about sex, as well as changing norms. Our own research at present is aimed at pinpointing the normative influences on talking about negotiating safer sex. There is much work still to be done. It may yet turn out that the most important variable in promoting safer sex is spreading the word about it.

ACKNOWLEDGMENTS

The project reported in this chapter was supported by a Commonwealth AIDS Research Grant to the authors; we also acknowledge the support of the Department of Psychology, The University of Queensland. We would like to acknowledge the contribution of our research colleagues, Deborah Terry, Ruth Hills, Perri Timmins, Anita Chauvin, and Andrew Ede, and to thank the editors of this book for their helpful comments on earlier drafts of the chapter.

REFERENCES

Abbott, S. (1987). *Talking about AIDS: A report on the issues of AIDS with young women.* Canberra, Australia: AIDS Action Council.

Ajzen, I. (1985). From intentions to actions: A theory of planned behavior. In J. Kuhl & J. Beckman (Eds.), *Action control* (pp. 11–19). New York: Springer.

Ajzen, I. (1988). *Attitudes, personality, and behaviour.* Buckingham: Open University Press.

Ajzen, I., & Fishbein, M. (1973). Attitudinal and normative variables as predictors of specific behaviors. *Journal of Personality and Social Psychology, 27,* 41–57.

Ajzen, I., & Fishbein, M. (1980). *Understanding attitudes and predicting social behavior.* Englewood Cliffs, NJ: Prentice-Hall.

Ajzen, I., & Madden, T. J. (1986). Prediction of goal-directed behavior: Attitudes, intentions, and perceived behavioral control. *Journal of Experimental Social Psychology, 22,* 453–474.

Anderson, N. H. (1967). Averaging model analysis of the set-size effect in impression formation. *Journal of Experimental Psychology, 75,* 158–165.

Andrews, R. P., & Kandel, D. B. (1979). Attitude and behavior: A specification of the contingent consistency hypothesis. *American Sociological Review, 44,* 298–310.

Bagozzi, R. P., & Schnedlitz, P. (1985). Social contingencies in the attitude model: A test of certain interaction hypotheses. *Social Psychology Quarterly, 48,* 366–373.

Bandura, A. (1989). Perceived self-efficacy in the exercise of control over AIDS infection. In W. M. Mays, G. W. Albee, & S. F. Schneider (Eds.), *Primary prevention of AIDS: Psychological approaches* (pp. 128–141). Newbury Park: Sage.

Bauman, L. J., & Siegel, K. (1987). Misperception among gay men of the risk for AIDS associated with their sexual behavior. *Journal of Applied Social Psychology, 17,* 329–350.

Becker, M. H., Drachman, R. H., & Kirscht, J. P. (1974). A new approach to explaining sick-role behavior in low-income populations. *American Journal of Public Health, 64*, 205–216.

Bentler, P. M., & Speckart, G. (1979). Models of attitude-behavior relations. *Psychological Review, 47*, 265–276.

Bentler, P. M., & Speckart, G. (1981). Attitudes 'cause' behaviors: A structural equations analysis. *Journal of Personality and Social Psychology, 40*, 226–238.

Budd, R. J. (1986). Predicting cigarette use: Models of attitude behavior relations. *Journal of Applied Social Psychology, 16*, 663–685.

Budd, R. J., & Spencer, C. P. (1985). Exploring the role of personal normative beliefs in the theory of reasoned action: The problem of discriminating between alternative path models. *European Journal of Social Psychology, 15*, 299–313.

Connell, R., Crawford, J., Kippax, S., Dowsett, G., Baxter, D., Watson, L., & Berg, R. (1989). Facing the epidemic: Changes in the sexual and social lives of gay and bisexual men in response to the AIDS crisis, and their implications for AIDS prevention strategies. *Social Problems, 36*, 384–402.

Connell, R., & Kippax, S. (1990). Sexuality in the AIDS crisis: Patterns of sexual practice and pleasure in a sample of Australian gay and bisexual men. *The Journal of Sex Research, 27*, 1–32.

Crawford, J., Kippax, S., & Tulloch, J. (1991). *Evaluation of national AIDS education campaigns.* Report to the Department of Community Services and Health, Canberra.

Crawford, J., Turtle, A., & Kippax, S. (1990). Student-favoured strategies for AIDS avoidance. *Australian Journal of Psychology, 42*, 123–137.

Davidson, A. R., & Jaccard, J. (1979). Variables that moderate the attitude-behavior relation: Results of a longitudinal survey. *Journal of Personality and Social Psychology, 37*, 1364–1376.

Davidson, A. R., Yantis, S., Norwood, M., & Montano, D. E. (1985). Amount of information about the attitude object and attitude-behavior consistency. *Journal of Personality and Social Psychology, 49*, 1184–1198.

Fazio, R. H., Powell, M. C., & Herr, P. M. (1983). Toward a process model of the attitude-behavior relation: Accessing one's attitude upon mere observation of the attitude object. *Journal of Personality and Social Psychology, 44*, 723–735.

Fazio, R. H., & Zanna, M. P. (1981). Direct experience and attitude-behavior consistency. In L. Berkowitz (Ed.), *Advances in experimental social psychology* (Vol. 14, pp. 161–202). New York: Academic Press.

Fishbein, M., & Ajzen, I. (1975). *Belief, attitude, intention, and behavior: An introduction to theory and research.* Reading, MA: Addison-Wesley.

Fishbein, M., & Middlestadt, S. E. (1987). Using the theory of reasoned action to develop educational interventions: Applications to illicit drug use. *Health Education Research, 2*, 361–371.

Fishbein, M., & Middlestadt, S. E. (1989). Using the theory of reasoned action as a framework for understanding and changing AIDS-related behaviors. In V. M. Mays, G. W. Albee, & S. F. Schneider (Eds.), *Primary prevention of AIDS: Psychological approaches* (pp. 93–110). Newbury Park: Sage.

Fisher, J. D. (1988). Possible effects of reference group-based social influence on AIDS-risk behavior and AIDS prevention. *American Psychologist, 43*, 914–920.

Fisher, J. D., & Fisher, W. A. (1990). *A general social psychological model for changing AIDS risk behavior.* Manuscript submitted for publication.

Fisher, W. A. (1984). Predicting contraceptive behavior among university men: The role of emotions and behavioral intentions. *Journal of Applied Social Psychology, 14*, 104–123.

Fisher, W. A. (1990). Understanding and preventing teenage pregnancy and sexually transmitted disease/AIDS. In J. Edwards, R. S. Tindale, L. Heath, & E. J. Posavac (Eds.), *Social influence processes and prevention* (pp. 71–101). New York: Plenum.

Fredericks, A. J., & Dossett, D. L. (1983). Attitude-behavior relations: A comparison of the Fishbein-Ajzen and the Bentler-Speckart models. *Journal of Personality and Social Psychology, 45,* 501–512.

Gallois, C., Kashima, Y., Hills, R., & McCamish, M. (1990, June). *Preferred strategies for safe sex: Relation to past and actual behaviour among sexually active men and women.* Paper presented at the sixth International Conference on AIDS, San Francisco.

Gallois, C., Kashima, Y., Terry, D., McCamish, M., Timmins, P., & Chauvin, A. (in press). Safe and unsafe sexual intentions and behavior: The effects of norms and attitudes. *Journal of Applied Social Psychology.*

Gallois, C., Timmins, P., McCamish, M., Terry, D., & Kashima, Y. (1991, April). *Perceived personal risk, information, and contact with AIDS: Relation to safe sexual practice.* Paper presented at the Twentieth Annual Meeting of Australian Social Psychologists, Ballarat, Victoria, Australia.

Gold, R. S., Skinner, M. J., Grant, P. J., & Plummer, D. C. (in press). Situational factors and thought processes associated with unprotected intercourse in gay men. *Psychology and Health.*

Grube, J. W., Morgan, M., & McGree, S. T. (1986). Attitudes and normative beliefs as predictors of smoking intentions and behaviours: A test of three models. *British Journal of Social Psychology, 25,* 81–93.

Heaven, P. C. L. (1987). Beliefs about the spread of the acquired immunodeficiency syndrome. *The Medical Journal of Australia, 147,* 272–274.

Kashima, Y., Gallois, C., Hills, R., & McCamish, M. (1991). *Intentions, past behaviour, future behaviour: When does intention to use a condom predict actual use?* Manuscript submitted for publication.

Kashima, Y., Gallois, C., & McCamish, M. (1991). *Conceptualising social influences in the theory of reasoned action: Effects of norms and partner on condom use intentions.* Manuscript submitted for publication.

Kashima, Y., & Kashima, E. (1988). Individual differences in the prediction of behavioral intentions. *Journal of Social Psychology, 128,* 711–720.

Kelly, J. A., St. Lawrence, J. S., Stevenson, L. Y., Diaz, Y. E., Hauth, A. C., Brasfield, T. L., Smith, J. E., Bradley, B. G., & Bahr, G. R. (1990, June). *Population-wide risk behavior reduction through diffusion of innovation following intervention with natural opinion leaders.* Paper presented at the sixth International Conference on AIDS, San Francisco.

Kilty, K. M. (1978). Attitudinal and normative variables as predictors of drinking behavior. *Journal of Studies of Alcohol, 39,* 1178–1194.

Kirscht, J. P., & Joseph, J. G. (1989). The health belief model: Some implications for behavior change, with reference to homosexual males. In V. M. Mays, G. W. Albee, & S. F. Schneider (Eds.), *Primary prevention of AIDS: Psychological approaches* (pp. 111–127). Newbury Park: Sage.

Liska, A. E. (1984). A critical examination of the causal structure of the Fishbein/Ajzen attitude-behavior model. *Social Psychology Quarterly, 47,* 61–74.

Manstead, A. S. R., Proffitt, C., & Smart, J. L. (1983). Predicting and understanding infant-feeding intentions and behavior: Testing the theory of reasoned action. *Journal of Personality and Social Psychology, 44,* 657–671.

McCamish, M., Cox, S., Frazer, I., & North, P. (1988, June). *Self-reported changes in sexual practices among gay and bisexual men as a result of AIDS awareness in a low-risk city.* Paper presented at the fourth International Conference on AIDS, Stockholm.

McCamish, M., Gallois, C., Arklay, A., & Wright, E. (1989). *Knowledge and beliefs about AIDS among students at The University of Queensland.* Report to the Queensland Department of Health, Brisbane.

McLaws, M.-L., Ross, M. W., Oldenberg, B., & Cooper, D. A. (1989, August). *Barriers to continued condom use.* Paper presented at the Australian Conference on Medical and Scientific Aspects of AIDS and HIV Infection, Sydney.
Middlestadt, S. E., & Fishbein, M. (1990, June). *Factors influencing experienced and inexperienced college women's intentions to tell their partners to use condoms.* Paper presented at the sixth International Conference on AIDS, San Francisco.
Morin, S. F., & Batchelor, W. (1984). Responding to the psychological crisis of AIDS. *Public Health Reports, 99,* 4–9.
Pagel, M. D., & Davidson, A. R. (1984). A comparison of three social-psychological models of attitude and behavioral plan: Prediction of contraceptive behavior. *Journal of Personality and Social Psychology, 47,* 517–523.
Peterson, C. C., & Peterson, J. L. (1987). Australian students' ratings of the importance of AIDS relative to other community problems. *Australian Journal of Sex, Marriage, and the Family, 8,* 194–200.
Puckett, S. B., & Bye, L. L. (1987). *The Stop-AIDS project: An interpersonal AIDS prevention plan.* Report to the San Francisco AIDS Foundation, San Francisco.
Rosenstock, I. M. (1974). The health belief model and preventative health behavior. *Health Education Monographs, 2,* 354–386.
Rosenthal, D., Moore, S., & Brumen, I. (1990). Ethnic group differences in adolescents' responses to AIDS. *Australian Journal of Social Issues, 3,* 220–239.
Ross, M. W. (1988). Prevalence of risk factors for human immunodeficiency virus infection in the Australian population. *Medical Journal of Australia, 1149,* 362–365.
Ross, M. W., & McLaws, M.-L. (in press). Normative beliefs about condoms are better predictors of use and intention to use than behavioral beliefs. *Health Education Research.*
Ross, M. W., Rigby, K., Rosser, B. R. S., Brown, M., & Anagnostou, P. (1990). The effect of a national campaign on attitudes towards AIDS. *AIDS Care, 2,* 339–346.
Schifter, D. B., & Ajzen, I. (1985). Intention, perceived control, and weight loss: An application of the theory of planned behavior. *Journal of Personality and Social Psychology, 49,* 843–851.
Schwartz, H. S., & Tessler, R. C. (1972). A test of a model for reducing measured attitude-behavior discrepancies. *Journal of Personality and Social Psychology, 24,* 225–236.
Siegel, K., & Gibson, W. (1988). Barriers to the modification of sexual behavior among heterosexuals at risk for acquired immunodeficiency syndrome. *New York State Journal of Medicine, 8,* 66–70.
Turtle, A. M., Ford, B., Habgood, R., Grant, M., Bekiaris, J., Constantinou, C., Macek, M., & Polyzoidis, H. (1989). AIDS-related beliefs and behaviours of Australian university students. *The Medical Journal of Australia, 150,* 371–376.
Waldby, C., Kippax, S., & Crawford, J. (1990). Theory in the bedroom: A report from Macquarie University AIDS and heterosexuality project. *Australian Journal of Social Issues, 3,* 177–185.
Weinstein, N. D. (1989). Perceptions of personal susceptibility to harm. In V. M. Mays, G. W. Albee, & S. F. Schneider (Eds.), *Primary prevention of AIDS: Psychological approaches* (pp. 142–167). Newbury Park: Sage.
Wilders, S., & MacCallum, M. (1990). *Research report: Women and AIDS.* Report to the Department of Community Services and Health, Canberra, Australia.
Wood, W. (1982). Retrieval of attitude-relevant information from memory: Effects on susceptibility to persuasion and on intrinsic motivation. *Journal of Personality and Social Psychology, 42,* 798–810.
Wright, B. (1990). *Student perceptions of AIDS: Seriousness and personal risk assessments.* Unpublished master's thesis, The University of Queensland, St. Lucia, Qld., Australia.
Wu, C., & Shaffer, D. R. (1987). Susceptibility of persuasive appeals as a function of source credibility and prior experience with the attitude object. *Journal of Personality and Social Psychology, 52,* 677–688.

CHAPTER THREE

A Compliance-Based Approach to the Study of Condom Use

Timothy Edgar
University of Maryland

In her book, *Erotic Wars,* Rubin (1990) quoted from an interview she conducted with a 36-year-old man on his feelings about sex. He said:

> Nothing makes you feel as . . . well, I don't know . . . alive, I'd guess you could say. You know, you feel kind of dead around the edges and you get up a good head of steam, and, wow, you're living man. (p. 99)

Certainly, he is not alone in his enthusiasm. Few, if any, other life activities bring people the kind of physical gratification and emotional emancipation as does sex. However, the AIDS crisis has created a situation where the activity that can make someone feel so alive can also lead to death. Fortunately, methods of AIDS prevention exist. One can make a number of safer-sex choices, but, short of abstinence, use of condoms is considered the most effective (Reiss & Leik, 1989).

A critical barrier to this safer-sex choice is communicating to one's sexual partner the desire to use a condom. Unlike other behaviors for the protection of one's health, condom use is not a unilateral practice. Unless one partner is completely naive to the realities of sex, condoms cannot be used unobtrusively. Agreement and cooperation are necessary conditions for completion of the precautionary behavior (Edgar, Hammond, & Freimuth, 1989). In order for a condom to be used, one person, at some level, must develop a behavioral goal and then enact a plan for expressing his or her wish. In other words, a successful attempt at compliance-gaining occurs. Communicating, however, about sex and activities related to sex is not a simple task for many individuals despite the fascination with the topic. As Foucault (1990) argued, in our public discourse "we talk more about sex than anything else; we set our minds to the task; we convince ourselves that we have never said enough on the topic" (p. 33). Yet, our ease with public discourse about sex does not necessarily match our level of comfort in private contexts.

The general purpose of this chapter is to better understand how individuals communicate to each other about using condoms. In particular, I examine the role of compliance-gaining in safe-sex situations. First, I present a model of condom use that includes a communication component. Second, I use Dillard's (1990) Goal-Driven Model of Interpersonal Influence as a framework for understanding why individuals do or do not use condoms. And, third, I review the literature on condom use and communication skills to show how persuasive skills function as vital interpersonal resources.

A MODEL OF CONDOM USE

Many researchers have tried to explain decisions people make about condom use (see Brafford & Beck, 1991; Bruce, Shrum, Trefethen, & Slovik, 1990; DeBuono, Zinner, Daamen, & McCormack, 1990; DiClemente, Forrest, Mickler, & Principal Site Investigators, 1990; Goodwin & Roscoe, 1988; Hebert, Bernard, de Man, & Farrar, 1989; Keeling, 1987). Typically, the focus of analysis is on the individual, either his or her personality characteristics or attitudes. Few researchers venture beyond the individual and investigate the interaction between partners (i.e., communication is missing from the models). Based on data in which individuals described their personal experiences in sexual encounters, we have developed a model that includes communication as a vital part of the process (Freimuth, Hammond, Edgar, McDonald, & Fink, in press). We surveyed 204 college students who had had a new sexual partner within the 12-month period prior to data collection, asking them to focus on their most recent experience of having sex for the first time with a new partner. They answered a series of open-ended questions related to interaction about the use of condoms and strategies to exert and resist influence. From this information we produced a three-stage model of condom use.

The first stage is an intention to use a condom (desire); the second stage, the initiation of a discussion with a partner about using a condom (initiate); and the third stage, actual use of a condom (use). Based on patterns of how the participants followed the three stages, we identified five types of individuals. Two of these groups are condom users and three are not. We called the first group of condom users in our typology *assertives*. They exhibit the "correct" attitude toward condoms, bring up the subject with their partners, and successfully enact the preventive behavior of using condoms. The other group of condom users follow an alternative pattern, non-desire, non-initiate, but use, and are called *compliers*. These individuals do not want to use a condom and do not initiate a discussion about condom use, but they do use one, presumably under pressure from an assertive partner. If partners of compliers do not initiate a discussion about condoms, it is unlikely that they would use protection.

Of the three groups of non-users of condoms, we labeled the first group *disinteresteds*. They do not want to use a condom and do not use one. Disinteresteds are probably the most resistant to change, although they may be converted by assertive partners. The other two patterns followed by non-users are called *passives* and *unsuccessfuls*. The passives want to use a condom but do not initiate a discussion about use, and end up not using one. The unsuccessfuls say they want to use a condom, initiate a discussion, but no condom is used.[1]

1. desire/initiate/use (assertives)
2. non-desire/non-initiate/use (compliers)
3. non-desire/non-initiate/non-use (disinteresteds)
4. desire/non-initiate/non-use (passives)
5. desire/initiate/non-use (unsuccessfuls)

Condom Use and Interpersonal Communication

The individuals in all five categories are of interest to the health communication scholar; however, a dyadic level of analysis is more appropriate and informative for some groups than others. In particular, disinteresteds profit most from analysis at the level of public communication. They present a great challenge for those who study health campaigns (see chapters by Freimuth, Salmon & Kroger, and Marková & Power, this volume). Not only do disinteresteds not use condoms, but also they have no desire to do so. The goal of the communication researcher should be to determine why the disinterested person lacks concern (e.g., insufficient knowledge of the problem or no personalization of risk) and then design and target messages that will prompt a change in attitude and subsequent action. This does not mean that the disinteresteds have no relevance to communication scholars who study messages at the dyadic level. The link, however, between the ultimate behavior of disinteresteds and inter-

---

[1]A sixth possible variation is desire/non-initiate/use, but because of the structure of the original questionnaire, we were unable to classify any respondents into this category. Like compliers, individuals who would fall into this classification are probably partners of assertives.

personal communication is not clear. Certainly, one can imagine at least two situations in which interpersonal communication is integral to the decision not to use a condom. In the first scenario, the final outcome for the disinterested individual is a result of the partner's interpersonal ineffectiveness. For example, the partner may desire to use a condom and conveys this wish, but the disinterested person refuses to acquiesce. A second viable portrait of interaction for the disinterested is one that he or she anticipates persuasive messages from the partner about condom use and actively tries to convince the partner that practicing safer sex is not a desirable option. It is just as possible, however, that communication about condoms plays no role at all for the disinterested individual. If he or she has a partner who shares the lack of desire to use condoms, then there may be no discussion of the issue.

The other four groups in our typology fall more clearly within the domain of the interpersonal communication researcher. By definition, communication about condom use must occur at some level in the interactions of three of the remaining four groups. We can assume that two types of individuals—assertives and compliers—are members of dyads in which the outcome is the result of a successful attempt at compliance. The assertives initiate discussion about condom use and achieve their desired goal. Obviously, their strategies for compliance are effective. The compliers show no initial interest in safer-sex practices, but yet they do use condoms. In order for this outcome to have occurred, the complier's partner must have indicated either verbally or nonverbally a desire to use a condom. The final group of individuals—passives—do not necessarily engage in discourse about safer sex. We know that the desire to use a condom is present, but because passives forego initiation of discussion about the topic and do not use condoms, it is very possible, if not probable, that the subject never is addressed by either partner. Still, passives present interpersonal researchers with a fascinating puzzle. Why do these individuals who want to practice safer sex not enact message strategies to attain their goal? Are there factors related to the particular dyad that inhibit attempts on the part of the passive person to gain compliance?

A MODEL OF INTERPERSONAL INFLUENCE

As a framework for understanding the role of compliance in safer-sex practices, I turn to Dillard's Goal-Driven Model of Interpersonal Influence (Dillard, 1990; Dillard, Segrin, & Hardin, 1989). I use the model to help explain why the assertives and compliers use condoms and unsuccessfuls and passives do not. In doing so, I refer to the literature on the relationship between communication skills and condom use.

Goals, Plans, and Action

In contrast to the trend of compliance-gaining research to focus on taxonomy development (Miller, Boster, Roloff, & Seibold, 1987), Dillard concentrated on process. The foundation of his model is a three-stage sequence of events—goals, planning, and action (GPA). According to Dillard (1990) *goals* are defined as "future states of affairs which an individual is committed to achieving or maintaining" (p. 43). In a given situation in which compliance is desired, two types of goals are simultaneously present: influence, or primary goals, and secondary goals. Influence goals drive the attempt at influence, whereas secondary goals function as a counterforce or inhibitors to the influence goal. In the case of sexual interaction, the wish to convince one's sexual partner to use a condom may function as the primary goal, whereas the desire to not interfere with the pleasure of lovemaking can serve as a secondary goal. The interplay between influence and secondary goals helps to determine an individual's subsequent plan and message output. At the point that secondary goals overwhelm primary goals an individual may abandon the influence attempt altogether.

The second stage in Dillard's model involves planning. More precisely, he uses the term *tactic plan* to refer to "a representation of a set of verbal and nonverbal actions that might modify the behavior of the target" (Dillard, 1990, p. 48). The development of plans, which can range in structure from simple to complex, may begin before or after one makes the final decision to engage in a compliance-gaining effort. Degree of complexity depends on the number and the sequence of elements and contingencies within the tactic plan. Dillard believes that planning involves two distinct activities: tactic plan generation and tactic plan selection. The former refers to the processes of retrieving and creating tactic plans. Each individual possesses a cognitive repertoire of plans from which to choose. Tactic plan selection relates to the ordering of plans.

The last stage of the model involves putting the plan into action. Dillard pointed out, however, that people often encounter at least two types of obstacles to plan implementation. First, some individuals do not have the necessary resources to complete a plan. Dillard (1990) provided the examples of people who lack sufficient evidence to support logic-based arguments or powerless individuals who use threats. Second, Dillard asserted those with limited cognitive capacities (either due to an individual difference or a situational factor) face difficulties when attempting to instantiate complex plans. In his own work, for instance, Dillard et al. (1989) found that arousal can inhibit the use of logic.

Inhibitors to Plans

Using the GPA sequence as a guide, we can start to account for individual behaviors and outcomes among the various groups. I begin my analysis with the passives because much of their behavior may be accounted for in what happens at the first stage. That is, many of them probably do not get beyond the formulation of the primary goal of wanting to use a condom. Dillard's treatment of secondary goals demonstrates how this can happen. As stated earlier, secondary goals often block or counteract influence goals. The passive individual may want to use a condom but feels constrained from pursuing the issue. A single secondary goal can inhibit pursuit of a primary goal or multiple secondary goals can operate simultaneously as a united force of constraint. Dillard and his colleagues (Dillard, 1990; Dillard et al., 1989) have identified five types of secondary goals. It is easy to imagine a scenario for how each one of these could counteract the primary goal of safer sex.

The first secondary goal Dillard described is an *identity goal*. This type of goal relates to one's sense of self. Identity goals stem from moral standards, life principles, and one's orientation toward personal conduct. For example, a passive individual who has concerns about the morality of premarital sex may want to use a condom. However, he or she may forego an attempt at persuasion because overt discussion about the event makes it too real. Indeed, Fisher, Byrne, and White (1983) have argued that adolescents with more conservative sexual values tend to use birth control less than their counterparts with a more liberal outlook toward sex. Their explanation for this pattern is that individuals in the former group avoid behaviors that make the sexual experience appear planned. By avoiding the use of contraceptives, the conservative adolescent can more easily convince him or herself that sex "just happened." Thus, the subsequent guilt will be less intense or nonexistent.

The second and third categories of secondary goals both focus on resources. *Relational resource goals* aim to protect one's relational assets (e.g., attention, affection, and support). If, for instance, a passive woman believes that asking her male partner to use a condom for protection against sexually transmitted diseases (STDs) might anger him and jeopardize the relationship, then she must choose which risk she can most afford to take. Does she risk damage to the relationship or does she take the chance of becoming infected with a disease? This type of secondary goal may be especially relevant in the initial stages of a relationship when uncertainty about both the present status and the future of the relationship is high. *Personal resource goals* pertain to physical, material, mental, and temporal assets. Many men and women believe, for example, that condoms diminish the physical pleasure of sex. As a result, a belief in the wisdom of condoms for disease prevention may be overshadowed by concerns for one's own sexual enjoyment. As Leishman (1987) has argued, "Even for many of those who worry about AIDS, the prospect of an orgasm in ten minutes eclipses any thought of the next twenty years of their lives" (p. 57).

The fourth type of secondary goal is an *arousal management goal.* This classification refers to an individual's attempt to maintain a comfortable psychological state. Many people feel uneasy with any direct discussion of sex. When sexual conversation leaps to the level of concern about one's life, then acceptable boundaries of comfort may be surpassed even further. An excerpt from an interview by Rubin (1990) of a 15-year-old female illustrates the point well. The girl described her nervous apprehensions about discussing condom use with her boyfriend: "A few times he's wanted to do it without anything, and I always think, next time that happens I'll tell him he can't, but then I can't make the words come out of my mouth" (p. 78).

The final category is labeled *interaction goals.* Here, one's concern is to impression manage. The individual wants to avoid behavior that might cause the target of persuasion to develop a negative opinion of him or her. In trying to get a partner to use a condom, many individuals will directly address anxieties about contracting AIDS. However, Collins (1990) found that a sexual partner who directly expresses a concern about AIDS often is perceived as uptight, weak, passive, geeky, and unattractive. Anyone worried about projecting this image probably will either develop an alternative plan for achieving the primary goal (i.e., getting the partner to use a condom) or, as in the case of many passives, completely retreat from the goal of safer sex.

Plan Implementation

Not all passives, however, necessarily terminate the compliance process at the first stage. Certainly, there are passives who develop plans but never enact them. This group of passives may best be understood by examining the planning and action stages of the Dillard model. Likewise, assertives, compliers, and unsuccessfuls differentiate based on contrasts within the final stages. Assertives (who are probably the partners for compliers) and unsuccessfuls are alike in that individuals in both groups have a goal of using a condom and, because they initiate discussion about the issue, we can assume that they develop a plan and attempt to put it into action. The difference is in the eventual outcome—assertives achieve their goal, whereas unsuccessfuls do not. Thus, we have individuals who generate plans but do not implement them, those who plan and implement unsuccessfully, others who plan and implement with success, and still others, despite their initial wishes, have plans successfully thrust upon them by their partners. The key question is: What occurs in the planning and action stages that separates the groups? The answer may lie in the actual or perceived resources that the individuals bring to the encounter.

Studies on Communication and Condom Use

Certainly, as Dillard pointed out, resources can take various forms. However, for the communication scholar the most important form of resource to analyze is the interactional resource. Specifically, I refer to the types of communication skills individuals possess that allow or deter them from successful enactment of their plans. Fortunately, there exists a body of literature, although limited, that provides clues about the kinds of skills that can be utilized as resources for putting plans for condom use into effective action. The drawback of the literature is that almost all of it is dependent on self-report. Due to the nature of the behavior under scrutiny, ethical considerations prevent direct or experimental observation. We can only rely on what subjects tell researchers about their behavior in private moments. However, despite the shortcomings, consistency exists within the literature. Regardless of the characteristics of the population under investigation (e.g., age, race, gender, area of country, sexual orientation), those who possess similar communication skills are more likely to use condoms in the appropriate situations.

Some of the published studies provide less direct evidence than others that communication proficiency discriminates between users and nonusers of condoms. This is because the earliest studies pre-date the advent of AIDS. Thus, the focus of investigation was not the prevention of HIV infection but birth control. The primary concern of researchers was to assess the relationship between communication behavior and a variety of contraceptive practices of which condom use was but one type.

Although they did not examine condom use specifically, Campbell and Barnlund (1977) did present preliminary evidence that one's ability to communicate skillfully may increase the likelihood that birth control will be used. They compared survey responses of 56 sexually active females residing in the San Francisco area. The researchers divided the subjects, who were predominantly White and lower middle class, into two groups of equal size. They labeled one group effective contraceptors (EC); the other group was called ineffective contraceptors (IC). Campbell and Barnlund categorized participants based on their responses to two questions: (a) I have had more than one unplanned pregnancy since 1963 (the date when oral contraceptives became widely available); and (b) I have never been pregnant.

Subjects also answered questions representing six measures of communication behavior:

1. a record of the amount of time subjects had spent talking to other people during a 3-day period;
2. Schutz' Firo-B measure of desire for inclusion, affection, and control in interpersonal interactions;
3. an interpersonal assessment of the ability to listen, empathize, handle anger, and express feelings and ideas;
4. a scale on the breadth and depth of self-disclosures to friends and family;
5. a test of body accessibility indicating the extent to which touch was used as a means of maintaining interpersonal contact; and
6. a defensive response scale that identified the preferred verbal responses in threatening or disturbing situations.

None of the questions directly asked about contraceptive-related communication with one's sexual partner(s).

Results indicated that ECs and ICs differed on several aspects of reported communication behavior. The ECs tended to be more frank and direct, more disclosive on all topics including sexuality issues, and more likely to have engaged in touching behavior with same sex friends. Also, ECs tended to respond defensively through humor and sarcasm, whereas ICs reported a proclivity for avoidance reactions when feeling threatened. Campbell and Barnlund felt that the results indicate that ICs tend to idealize relationships. The ICs may want to believe that contraceptive issues will take care of themselves and do not require any form of discussion or negotiation with one's partner. The results also suggest that ECs are more comfortable with their own sexuality.

Polit-O'Hara and Kahn (1985) also examined general communication ability in relation to birth control practices. Their approach differed, however, from Campbell and Barnlund in two fundamental ways. First, Polit-O'Hara and Kahn developed a sample comprised of couples. They interviewed 83 unmarried couples from Boston. All of the couples had been sexually active for at least 2 months prior to the interview, and all female members of the couples were between the ages of 15 and 18 and not pregnant. Second, their measure of communicative ability was not based solely on the participants' own assessment of skill. During the interviews, the researchers asked subjects about the frequency with which they communicated with their partners, the quality of the communication, and the range of topics discussed with partners. Judges later read the responses of both partners and assigned communication effectiveness ratings to each member of the couple. Results showed a moderate negative relationship ($r = -.37$) between communication effectiveness and risky behavior for all subjects. That is, the more individuals were perceived to be ineffective communicators, the more likely they were to engage in sex without protection.

The first systematic investigation of communication behavior as it relates specifically to condom use was undertaken by Cvetkovich and Grote (1981). Like the other research teams, Cvetkovich and Grote compared the communication abilities of users and non-users of contraception; however, they also assessed differences based on the type of preferred birth control. They interviewed 87 sexually active female high school students in the state of Washington. The interviews focused on the participants' role-taking skills and on self-disclosure behavior related to personal concerns, male–female relationships, home and family issues, and school. Also, a single bipolar question asked if the individual had discussed birth control with her partner prior to her sexual debut. Subjects who tended to use condoms not only had higher communication abilities than those who used no form of birth control, but they also reported greater skill than those who regularly used oral contraceptive.

A study by Ross (1988) also suggested that condom use is associated with communication skill. Although he did not specifically ask his gay male participants ($N = 148$) if they used condoms, he did measure their general attitudes toward condoms. Also, he used an adjective check to assess general behavioral and personality characteristics. Ross found that participants with positive attitudes toward condoms tended to view themselves as more assertive, interpersonally effective, confident, and goal attainers.

Catania et al. (1989) investigated the relationship between communication and condom use by surveying 114 female adolescents attending a family planning clinic in California. They specifically asked about communication with sexual partners through the use of two scales. The first one was more general in its approach. The scale measured the individual's perceived overall quality of sexual communication with primary partners. The scale contained items such as "My main partner really cares what I think about sex." The other measure was a single-item scale that assessed attempts to achieve compliance. The question asked the participants to indicate how often in the last 2 months they had requested that their main sexual partners use condoms during intercourse. These two variables were among the 10 used in a regression analysis to predict condom use. Only the compliance-related variable and enjoyment of condoms were significant predictors. Overall quality of sexual communication was not significant.

In our own work, we have attempted to identify the most common types of strategies individuals use to persuade a partner to use a condom and to assess the differences between condom users and non-users in their perceptions of these strategies (Edgar, Freimuth, Hammond, McDonald, & Fink, in press). In the same survey in which we obtained open-ended responses about actual past behavior, we also developed scenarios that contained hypothetical discussions between partners about condom usage. Two lines of dialogue were given in each scenario. The first statement represented an attempt to resist the partner, whereas the second statement was a strategy aimed at countering the resistance. Respondents indicated how likely they were to respond in the same way if confronted with a similar situation, and they assessed how persuasive they thought the strategy would be with a resistant partner of the opposite sex in their same age group.

The strategies used in the scenarios closely followed the distinctions made by Witteman and Fitzpatrick (1986) in their Verbal Interaction Compliance-Gaining Scheme (VICS). The types of strategies were:

1. *Me*—the force for compliance comes from within the persuader;
2. *You*—the force for compliance comes from within the target of compliance;
3. *Activity*—the force to comply focuses on the activity itself;
4. *Us*—the force to comply comes from the relationship between the two people involved;
5. *External*—the force to comply comes from a source outside the immediate relationship;
6. *Power (Reward)*—influence derives from the exertion of control when the persuader can reward the target of compliance;
7. *Power (Punishment)*—influence derives from the exertion of control when the persuader can punish the target of compliance;
8. *Direct*—the message is a straightforward request for compliance.

We also included a scenario in which the counter resistance message was a lie; a strategy of *deception* does not appear on the VICS. Two versions of each of the scenarios were created, one for males and the other for females (see the appendix).

A comparison of the strategy ratings between users and non-users of condoms revealed a tendency for condom users of both sexes to prefer messages that focus on health concerns rather than on giving or receiving sexual pleasure. In the male group, condom users said they are more likely than non-users to employ You and Power (punishment) strategies. Likewise, female condom users saw You strategies as more persuasive than non-users and viewed Power (punishment) strategies as more persuasive and more likely to be used.

Both the Power (punishment) and You strategies stress a concern for health. The former tacitly emphasizes protection of one's own health ("no condom, no sex"); the latter communicates consideration for the health of the target of compliance ("I care about you very much and don't want anything to happen to you"). In each case, the persuader implicitly displaces his or her own sexual needs to achieve the desired outcome.

Summary.   In summary, the results of these studies indicate that individuals who use condoms tend to be skillful communicators by most standards. Apparently, they are more assertive, more comfortable with higher levels of disclosure, more adept at managing conflict, and more empathic. One interpretation of these results is that compliance-gaining plans related to condom use are difficult to enact effectively unless one has a high degree of communicative skill. Perhaps these individuals meet with success because their superior communication abilities provide them with the necessary resources to develop more sophisticated initial plans for compliance and to generate workable contingencies when they meet with resistance. In other words, they are able to get their partners to use condoms because they can create the best strategies.

Other evidence, however, suggests that this conclusion is misleading. The latter interpretation rests on two basic assumptions. One is that a large number of attempts to convince a partner to use a condom are met with active resistance; the other is that there exists a set of "best" strategies that are more workable than others. Data exist that implies that both assumptions are either erroneous or overstated at the very least. In regard to the first assumption, our own findings indicate that resistance to a request to use a condom may be the exception instead of the rule (Edgar et al., in press). When participants in the study described their own experiences with discussion about condoms, very few recounted episodes in which a negotiation process took place. There was little evidence that partners who were asked to use a condom attempted to persuade the requestor otherwise. At first glance, this finding seems incongruent with our typology of condom users and non-users. Indeed, we identified unsuccessfuls as a primary category of individuals. They initiated discussion with their partners but no condom was used. However, most were unable to accomplish their primary goal not because they lacked the necessary communicative resources, but rather because they experienced a shortage of a crucial physical resource (i.e., the condom). Almost all of the unsuccessfuls did not use condoms due to the fact that none were available. Baffi, Schroeder, Redican, and McCluskey (1989) also found that the assumption of widespread resistance may be unfounded. Although a large proportion of their sample of college students said that they preferred not to use condoms, 83% reported at the same time that they would not object if their partners made the suggestion.[2]

Our data also called into question the second assumption that some strategies are more effective than others. Although condom users in our study gave higher persuasibility ratings to certain strategy types under hypothetical conditions, their reports on actual behavior suggested that the particular strategy choice tends to be inconsequential. In situations in which a condom was used, no one strategy or group of strategies increased the odds of success. There were preferences for strategy selection. For instance, female initiators relied primarily on a Direct message or a Power (punishment) strategy (i.e., "no condom, no sex"), whereas male initiators frequently chose a more nonverbal approach (i.e., putting the condom on without verbal discussion). Still, the strategy types least utilized produced comparable compliance responses.

Perhaps the key communication issue in understanding condom use is not the basic skills per se that individuals possess but rather their fundamental perceptions and beliefs about the importance of skill level for successful interpersonal influence. Consider, for instance, a female who has serious doubts about her communication skills related to compliance-gaining. She sees herself as not very assertive, generally feels uncomfortable with indepth disclosure about sexual issues, tends to avoid conflict when possible, and believes that her repertoire of persuasive strategies is very limited. As she enters a sexual liaison with her boyfriend, she desires that they practice safer sex. Because in her mind the only plan that she can generate is a simple, direct request, she feels that she does not have a "good" plan for action. If he does not acquiesce immediately, she has no alternative plan at her disposal. As a result of her assessment of the situation, she foregoes any attempt at compliance. In reality, is her pessimistic view warranted? Probably not. The concern then becomes to find ways in which to change such a person's perception of the situation. The solution to this puzzle may be found through communication skills training. The goal of the training would not necessarily be to produce individuals who can create sophisticated plans to meet any situation. Instead, the goal would be to provide people with a variety of plans so that they feel more confident about their chances for success. A perceived increase in communicative resources may prompt the individual to take the all important first step even though the variety of

---

[2]I do not want to minimize the frustrations an individual faces in those instances when resistance does occur. Certainly, there are occasions in which a clear power differential between partners leads to uncompromising stances. See Fullilove, Fullilove, Haynes, and Gross (1990) for examples of this pattern of interaction. Also, Metts and Fitzpatrick address the issue in the previous chapter.

plans at his or her disposal are not necessarily needed and probably will not be used.

Providing Communication Resources

There are a few published studies that provide some information about the efficacy of communication training related to safer sex. As with the self-report studies discussed previously, the earliest experimental work highlighting the relationship between communication skills and condom use comes from the birth control literature. Although they did not directly address the issue of condom use, Schinke, Gilchrist, and Blythe (1980) demonstrated that individuals can be trained to improve their sexually related compliance-gaining skills. Eighteen females between the ages of 14 and 17 participated in their experiment. At the time of the study, almost all of the subjects either had at least one child or were pregnant. Prior to experimental manipulation, the researchers videotaped subjects while they interacted with a confederate in a hypothetical scenario. The confederate played the role of a "date" trying to convince the female to have sex with him. The females attempted to enact strategies that would counteract his demands. After the initial roleplay, half of the subjects received training in interpersonal skills, while the other half took part in group discussions about the difficulties of interpersonal communication. All participants then role-played the same scenario with a confederate.

Analysis of the post-manipulation videotapes revealed that those who received training differed significantly in their communicative behavior from those who only took part in group discussions. The former group displayed greater eye contact, made more "I" statements, explicitly said "no" to role-play partners, communicated more direct refusals, and allowed less time to elapse between their partners' attempts at compliance and their own responses. Another key finding was that individuals in the training group reported that they felt more in control of their lives. As argued earlier, this sense of control or increased confidence may be the most important factor in precipitating plan implementation.

A study that specifically focused on communication about condom use was conducted by Solomon and DeJong (1989). Their experiment included a sample (N = 103) comprised of patients at an STD clinic in Boston. A large majority of the participants were African-American males who had never or almost never used condoms prior to their visit to the clinic.

Rather than provide direct skill instruction as did Schinke and his colleagues, Solomon and DeJong utilized a drama-based method (see Solomon & DeJong, 1986) in which subjects in an intervention group watched a soap opera-style videotape called "Let's Do Something Different" (Solomon & Nelson, 1986). The main character, Diane, is a young African-American heterosexual female who has had two cases of gonorrhea and most recently has been treated for pelvic inflammatory disease. Diane interacts in three distinct scenes with her brother, a girlfriend, and finally her boyfriend, Justin. Both the brother and girlfriend encourage her to use a condom when she and Justin have sex. The girlfriend goes a step further by offering advice, although minimal, on how to talk to Justin about the issue. She tells Diane that she should just slip the condom on him and then talk about it afterward.

Although she receives limited advice about communication, Diane does employ a variety of compliance-gaining strategies during her interaction with Justin. For example, early in the interaction Diane uses a Me message by focusing attention on her own health:

Diane: I mean, we've got to do something different.
Justin: Hmmm, okay. I'm into different.
Diane: That's not what I mean. This is serious . . . I can't afford to get sick again.

Later she relies on outside sources (External message) to make her case:

Justin: Guess what? It's all cleared up baby.
Diane: Wait, wait. Look, it says right here (as she reads a pamphlet), multiple cases of PID, that's pelvic inflammatory disease, can result in sterility. Do you know what that means? I wouldn't be able to have kids.

And finally, Diane tries to convince Justin that she will be able to provide physical pleasure for him despite the presence of the condom (Power [Reward] message):

Justin: Yeah, but I don't want to feel this rubber, baby. I want to feel you.
Diane: Baby, you'll feel me. I promise. And, uh, what do you say I put this on you? (she hands him a condom)

The dependent measure for the experiment was one open-ended question that asked: "If a person wants to convince his/her partner to use condoms, what are some things that person could do or say?" (Solomon & DeJong, 1989, p. 454). In the nonintervention group, 52% could not provide an answer, and only 8% were able to produce more than one strategy. Participants in the intervention group completed the task with greater ease. Although 22% still could not answer the question after watching the videotape, 24% wrote more than one strategy. The most frequently listed strategies included: arguing that condoms could be fun and did not have to diminish sexual pleasure and vetoing the sex act. Interestingly, Diane never used the latter strategy in the videotape. She did not directly threaten to withhold sex if her partner refused to comply.

Unfortunately, neither Schinke et al. (1980) nor Solomon and DeJong (1989) had data about how the learned behaviors translate into situations that are not hypothetical. That is, when confronted with a similar scenario in real life, are individuals able to enact the appropriate behaviors, or do the pressures and constraints of the moment negate what individuals have learned?

This important question has been answered in part by a research team working with a gay male population. Kelly, St. Lawrence, Hood, and Brasfield (1989) attempted to alter the communication behavior (and subsequently the sexual practices) of a group of sexually active gay males in Mississippi. All subjects in the predominantly White sample ($N = 104$) participated in eight role-play situations with a confederate. The role-play scenarios involved circumstances in which either the hypothetical partner tries to pressure the individual into having unsafe sex or proposes a sexual encounter that might require further discussion or negotiation (e.g., suggesting that the two first get to know each other better or declining the sexual advance). The men listened to the scenarios on audiotape then responded to a series of live prompts provided by the confederate. The researchers audiotaped the responses.

An experimental group later received assertiveness training dealing with three behavioral aspects: initiating precoital discussion with a partner about one's commitment to safer-sex practices, counteracting pressures to engage in unsafe practices, and declining immediate sexual advances from someone they first might like to know better. For instance, when they encountered situations in which partners pressured the men to engage in high-risk practices, participants were instructed "to acknowledge the partner's wish but to firmly refuse the partner's unsafe request, to provide a reason for the refusal, and to suggest an alternative that would not create risk" (p. 62). Group facilitators gave feedback to participants about their enactment of the skills and encouraged the men to utilize the skills in actual situations. In subsequent training sessions the participants reported on their assertiveness behavior and received additional information on relational strategies and on ways to express affection in a nonsexual manner.

After the training, both the experimental and control groups reported on their sexual practices over a 4-week period, and they participated again in the role-plays. Judges scored the postintervention tapes based on their assessment of the participants' overall effectiveness. They defined an effective response as one that would prevent the practice of unsafe behaviors. Results showed that the experimental group exhibited significantly greater skill than the control group in handling casual propositions and coercions to engage in risky behaviors. Also, experimental participants were more likely to acknowledge a partner's desires, give reasons for refusals, verbally refuse to practice unsafe sex, give reasons for the refusals, state why safety was important, and verbally provide suggestions for lower risk behavioral alternatives. Kelly et al. (1989) also found that men in the experimental group reported reduced frequency of unprotected sex and increased use of condoms. In a follow-up study employing the same design with a much smaller sample size ($N = 15$), Kelly, St. Lawrence, Betts, Brasfield, and Hood (1990) identified a similar pattern of behavior.[3]

Summary. Collectively, all three studies provide evidence that, at least on a short-term basis, one's persuasive repertoire can be enhanced through appropriate skills training. In the future, health communication researchers should follow the lead of Kelly and his associates by gathering data on real-life interactions. Also, further study is needed to determine how individuals perceive and respond to their new skills. Most importantly, researchers must determine at what point individuals view skills acquisition not just as an exercise in dialogue memorization but as a dynamic resource that enables them to implement desired plans. The solution to the puzzle may only come through longitudinal work.

CONCLUSION

This chapter has shown how a model of the compliance-gaining process is a useful theoretical hook for analyzing sexual interactions and the use of condoms. This framework is especially useful for understanding why a person would or would not view condom use as an important goal and why one would pursue particular plans for achieving the desired goal. Although the study of compliance-gaining does not answer all questions about communication and safer-sex practices (see Adelman, this volume), it does fill in many gaps in our knowledge about this important issue.

---

[3]Although the outcome highlights the vital role of communication activity, Kelly and his associates have acknowledged that other factors in their design (e.g., basic AIDS education) may have accounted for behavioral change (Kelly et al., 1989). Thus, they could not assess the relative contribution of the communication training.

APPENDIX

Hypothetical Scenarios (Female Version)

Scenario 1—Me
Male: "I know I'm OK (disease-free); I haven't had sex with anyone in months."
Female: "I'm glad you told me that, and as far as I know I'm OK, too. But I'm not taking any chances with my life."

Scenario 2—Power (Reward)
Male: "I'll lose my hard-on by the time I stop to put this on."
Female: "If you use one, I promise you I'm going to make you feel so good that there's no way that's going to happen."

Scenario 3—You
Male: "I hate condoms."
Female: "I understand what you're saying, but an infection isn't so great either. Let's try to work this out because I care about you very much and don't want anything to happen to you."

Scenario 4—Deception
Male: "Why do we need to use a condom? I wouldn't give you an infection."
Female: "I'm not concerned about an infection. I want to use it because I'm not using any form of birth control." (This is a lie; she is on the Pill.)

Scenario 5—External
Male: "This is insulting! Do you think I'm gay or something?"
Female: "No, I don't, but being gay has nothing to do with it. I've heard that everyone is at risk and should use condoms."

Scenario 6—Power (Punishment)
Male: "Let's do it just this once without a condom."
Female: "If you're not going to use a condom then we're not going to have sex at all."

Scenario 7—Activity
Male: "I can't feel a thing when I wear a condom. It's like wearing a raincoat in the shower."
Female: "Even if you lose some sensation you'll still have plenty left. Besides, don't you think it will be a real turn-on for you if you let me put it on for you?"

Scenario 8—Us
Male: "I don't want to do this. It destroys the romantic atmosphere."
Female: "I hope that we're attracted to each other enough for us to stay in the mood."

Scenario 9—Direct
Male: "You don't want me to use this, do you?" (the female has just handed him a condom)
Female: "Yes, I want you to use it."

Hypothetical Scenarios (Male Version)

Scenario 1—Me
Female: "I know I'm OK (disease-free); I haven't had sex with anyone in months."
Male: "I'm glad you told me that, and as far as I know I'm OK, too. But I'm not taking any chances with my life."

Scenario 2—Power (Reward)
Female: "By the time you put it on, I'll be out of the mood."
Male: "If you let me use one, I promise you I'm going to make you feel so good that there's no way that's going to happen."

Scenario 3—You
Female: "I hate condoms."
Male: "I understand what you're saying, but an infection isn't so great either. Let's try to work this out because I care about you very much and don't want anything to happen to you."

Scenario 4—Deception
Female: "Why do we need to use a condom? I wouldn't give you an infection."
Male: "I'm not concerned about an infection. I like to use condoms because when I use them I can go longer without coming." (This is a lie; he really is concerned about an infection.)

Scenario 5—External
Female: "What's the problem? Are you gay or something?"
Male: "No, I'm not, but that doesn't make any difference. I've heard that everyone is at risk and should use condoms."

Scenario 6—Power (Punishment)
Female: "Let's do it just this once without a condom."
Male: "If we're not going to use a condom then we're not going to have sex at all."

Scenario 7—Activity
Female: "I think using condoms makes sex less exciting."
Male: "It doesn't have to be that way. Don't you think it will be a real turn-on for you if you put it on me?"

Scenario 8—Us
Female: "I don't want to use a condom. It destroys the romantic atmosphere."
Male: "I hope that we're attracted to each other enough for us to stay in the mood."

Scenario 9—Direct
Female: "You aren't going to use a condom, are you?" (as he starts to take one out of the package)
Male: "Yes, I want us to use one."

REFERENCES

Baffi, C. A., Schroeder, K. K., Redican, K. J., & McCluskey, L. (1989). Factors influencing selected heterosexual male college students' condom use. *Journal of American College Health, 38,* 137–141.

Brafford, L. J., & Beck, K. H. (1991). Development and validation of the condom use self-efficacy scale for college students. *Journal of American College Health, 39,* 219–225.

Bruce, K. E., Shrum, J. C., Trefethen, C., & Slovik, L. F. (1990). Students' attitudes about AIDS, homosexuality, and condoms. *AIDS Education and Prevention, 2,* 220–234.

Campbell, B. K., & Barnlund, D. C. (1977). Communication style: A clue to unplanned pregnancy. *Medical Care, 15,* 181–186.

Catania, J. A., Coates, T. J., Greenblatt, R. M., Dolcini, M. M., Kegeles, S. M., Puckett, S., Corman, M., & Miller, J. (1989). Predictors of condom use and multiple partnered sex among sexually active adolescent women: Implications for AIDS-related health interventions. *Journal of Sex Research, 4,* 514–524.

Collins, B. E. (1990, May). *Identity processes in the negotiation of safer sex.* Paper presented at the Conference on Negotiating Safer Sex, San Diego.

Cvetkovich, G., & Grote, B. (1981). Psychosocial maturity and teenage contraceptive use: An investigation of decision-making and communication skills. *Population and Environment, 4,* 211–226.

DeBuono, B. A., Zinner, S. H., Daamen, M., & McCormack, W. M. (1990). Sexual behavior of college women in 1975, 1986, and 1989. *New England Journal of Medicine, 322,* 821–825.

DiClemente, R. J., Forrest, K. A., Mickler, S., & Principal Site Investigators. (1990). College students' knowledge and attitudes about AIDS and changes in HIV-preventive behaviors. *AIDS Education and Prevention, 2,* 201–212.

Dillard, J. P. (1990). A goal-driven model of interpersonal influence. In J. P. Dillard (Ed.), *Seeking compliance: The production of interpersonal influence messages* (pp. 41–56). Scottsdale, AZ: Gorsuch-Scarisbrick.

Dillard, J. P., Segrin, C., & Hardin, J. M. (1989). Primary and secondary goals in the production of interpersonal influence messages. *Communication Monographs, 56,* 19–38.

Edgar, T., Freimuth, V. S., Hammond, S. L., McDonald, D., & Fink, E. L. (in press). Strategic sexual communication: Condom use resistance and response. *Health Communication.*

Edgar, T., Hammond, S. L., & Freimuth, V. S. (1989). The role of the mass media and interpersonal communication in promoting AIDS-related behavioral change. *AIDS and Public Policy Journal, 4,* 3–9.

Fisher, W. A., Byrne, D., & White, L. A. (1983). Sex without contraception. In D. Byrne & W. A. Fisher (Eds.), *Adolescents, sex, and contraception* (pp. 207–239). Hillsdale, NJ: Lawrence Erlbaum Associates.

Foucault, M. (1990). *The history of sexuality: An introduction* (Vol. 1) (R. Hurley, Trans.). New York: Vintage Books. (Original work published 1976)

Freimuth, V. S., Hammond, S. L., Edgar, T., McDonald, D., & Fink, E. L. (in press). Factors explaining intent, discussion, and use of condoms in first-time sexual encounters. *Health Education Research: Theory and Practice.*

Fullilove, M. T., Fullilove, R. E., Haynes, K., & Gross, S. (1990). Black women and AIDS prevention: A view towards understanding the gender rules. *Journal of Sex Research, 27,* 47–64.

Goodwin, M. P., & Roscoe, B. (1988). AIDS: Students' knowledge and attitudes at a midwestern university. *Journal of American College Health, 36,* 214–222.

Hebert, Y., Bernard, J., de Man, A. F., & Farrar, D. (1989). Factors related to the use of condoms among French-Canadian university students. *Journal of Social Psychology, 129,* 707–709.

Keeling, R. P. (1987). Risk communication about AIDS in higher education. *Science, Technology, and Human Values, 12,* 3–27.

Kelly, J. A., St. Lawrence, J. S., Betts, R., Brasfield, T. L., & Hood, H. V. (1990). A skills-training group intervention model to assist persons in reducing risk behaviors for HIV infection. *AIDS Education and Prevention, 2,* 24–35.

Kelly, J. A., St. Lawrence, J. S., Hood, H. V., & Brasfield, T. L. (1989). Behavioral intervention to reduce AIDS risk activities. *Journal of Consulting and Clinical Psychology, 57,* 60–67.

Leishman, K. (1987, February). Heterosexuals and AIDS. *The Atlantic Monthly,* pp. 39–58.

Miller, G., Boster, F., Roloff, M., & Seibold, D. (1987). MBRS rekindled: Some thoughts on compliance gaining in interpersonal settings. In M. E. Roloff & G. R. Miller (Eds.), *Interpersonal processes: New directions in communication research* (pp. 89–116). Newbury Park, CA: Sage.

Polit-O'Hara, D., & Kahn, J. R. (1985). Communication and contraceptive practices in adolescent couples. *Adolescence, 20,* 33–43.

Reiss, I. L., & Leik, R. K. (1989). Evaluating strategies to avoid AIDS: Number of partners versus use of condoms. *Journal of Sex Research, 4,* 411–433.

Ross, M. W. (1988). Personality factors that differentiate homosexual men with positive and negative attitudes toward condom use. *New York State Journal of Medicine, 88,* 626–628.

Rubin, L. B. (1990). *Erotic wars: What happened to the sexual revolution?* New York: Farrar, Straus, & Giroux.

Schinke, S. P., Gilchrist, L. D., & Blythe, B. J. (1980). Role of communication in the prevention of teenage pregnancy. *Health and Social Work, 5,* 54–60.

Solomon, M. Z., & DeJong, W. (1986). Recent sexually transmitted disease prevention efforts and their implications for AIDS health education. *American Journal of Public Health, 79,* 453–458.

Solomon, M. Z., & DeJong, W. (1989). Preventing AIDS and other STDs through condom promotion: A patient education intervention. *Health Education Quarterly, 13,* 301–316.

Solomon, M. Z. (Producer), & Nelson, D. (Director). (1986). *Let's do something different* [Videotape]. Newton, MA: Education Development Center.

Witteman, H., & Fitzpatrick, M. A. (1986). Compliance-gaining in marital interaction: Power bases, processes, and outcomes. *Communication Monographs, 53,* 130–143.

CHAPTER FOUR

Healthy Passions:
Safer Sex as Play

Mara B. Adelman
Northwestern University

> *It's easy to take sex far too seriously and miss the joy of an elemental aspect of the human experience which lies at the intersection where the sublime meets the ridiculous.*
>
> —Burt (1990–1991, p. 12)

If AIDS has prompted an age of sexual caution, it has also generated an era of sexual invention. The loss of abandonment has now become the parent of invention, fueling those that seek to recapture the "pure presentness" (Sontag, 1989) that once pervaded the sexual encounter. In the search for alternatives in these cautionary times, Julia Kristeva observed that "there is the possibility of discovering new erogenous zones, the arousal of tenderness, and (at last) the erotic use of speech" (in Chapple & Talbot, 1989, p. 345). If so, then we must seek to understand the various genres of discourse that sexual partners use to pursue safer sex, enabling them to sustain passion while also ensuring physical well-being.

Understanding safer-sex discourse involves the study of metaphor, figures of speech that encode much of the way we think about a certain subject. Currently, the most prominent metaphor for the study of safer-sex communication is negotiation. In this chapter I critique the metaphor of safer sex as "negotiation" and offer the metaphor of "play" for understanding the improvisational side of this discourse. After outlining the incongruent tensions embodied in safer-sex practices, I identify several functions of play in facilitating sexual communication and in resolving the incongruities. Literature from diverse disciplines are used to illustrate these functions, followed by a play analysis of couples discussing safer sex. Finally, I conclude with implications for taking play seriously in sex education curriculum and in media representations of sexual encounters.

THE METAPHORS OF NEGOTIATION AND PLAY

Metaphors are powerful figures of speech that focus our attention on points of comparison, illuminating certain aspects of human phenomena to the exclusion of others (Lakoff & Johnson, 1980). Apart from serving as explanatory devices, metaphors also embody prescriptive elements. Morgan (1986) referred to these elements as the "injunction of the metaphor—systematic ways of thinking about how we can or should act in a given situation" (p. 331). By structuring thought through images, metaphors shape our social construction, scholarly theorizing, and empirical research of reality (see Koestler, 1964, chapter XVII; Sarbin, 1986). Such is the case in explaining safer-sex talk.

Safer Sex as Negotiation

Communication research on sex and safer sex tends to be modeled on the metaphor of negotiation. A recent conference entitled, "Negotiating Safer Sex: Social Science Theory and Research" suggests the prominence of this metaphor (Krier, 1990). Further support of this metaphor can be found in works on sex and safer-sex communication that focus on such aspects as influence strategies (Edgar & Fitzpatrick, 1988; Edgar, Freimuth, Hammond, McDonald, & Fink, in press; McCormick, 1979), scripts (LaPlante, McCormick, & Brannigan, 1980; Simon & Gagnon, 1988), and power and goals (see Metts & Cupach, 1989 for review; also see chapters by Edgar and Metts & Fitzpatrick, this volume). Apart from their literal or operational definitions, this focus suggests a highly scripted, rule-governed, premeditative, goal-driven account of the sexual encounter. The metaphor is understandably appealing to social scientists because it emphasizes control and management of the interaction. This emphasis is closely aligned with the highly prized outcomes of a positivist paradigm for research—to control and predict human behavior.

However, the metaphor seems glaringly out of sync when one tries to imagine actual people lying down and negotiating their sex lives. Quite frankly, it lacks "emotive potential," an ability to evoke or satisfy the particular emotions (Koestler, 1964). In this case, the image of negotiation does little to evoke emotions associated with sensuality and sexuality. Perhaps this absence of emotive potential is only an aesthetic and pragmatic critique rather than a methodological one. Nonetheless, sex as negotiation does not appeal to, much less reveal, the senses that often sustain lovers.

When applied to intimate relationships, the negotiation metaphor suggests a highly bracketed activity, something separate from the ongoing flow of social conversation. Seckman and Couch (1989) argued that the act of negotiation involves people taking "time out" while they work on their relationship. This may be problematic for sustaining mutual sexual pleasure. According to Davis (1983), any activity during the sexual encounter that may be perceived as taking time out can be highly disruptive to escalating sexual excitement, forcing partners back into the realm of everyday concerns. In terms of the sexual encounter, negotiating safer sex as a ground rule for intercourse suggests that couples bracket this discussion from the lasciviousness of the moment, creating a dysrhythmia that "may halt the sensual slide after it has begun to accelerate" (Davis, 1983, p. 64).

Rather than a product of explicit bargaining, the mutual agreements achieved prior to safer-sex encounters may be more likely to involve innuendo, allusion, and tacit understanding. Due to the taboo of sex talk in romantic relationships (Baxter & Wilmont, 1985), nonexplicit agreements between lovers may be preferable to explicit verbal contracts. These agreements, often coded through nonverbal channels, are similar to Strauss' (1978) notion of "silent bargains," where "limits are tested and stretched, usually without actual negotiations. . . . Testing is often uncalculated and its cues are so gestural" (pp. 224–225).

Likewise, defining such nonexplicit agreements as *negotiation* tests the limits of the word itself. If the term *negotiation* is used so broadly as to encompass all forms of human interaction that facilitate mutual understanding, then the term becomes almost synonymous with communication and is in danger of losing its analytic power (Seckman & Couch, 1989; Strauss, 1978).

In short, the metaphor "safer sex as negotiation" suggests an experience that is controlling and explicit. In fact, sexual activity tends to be improvisational, suspended, and unpredictable. Improvisation is a more likely recourse for couples lacking a routine or script for practicing safer sex, especially for couples in newly formed sexual relationships. In part, the absence of a well-defined plan or script may force couples to improvise as they seek mutual understanding regarding condom use.

Because sexual encounters must adapt to the "practical circumstances" of the situation (e.g., need for privacy, timing, contraception), these practicalities present innumerable opportunities for improvisation (Ruelfi, 1985). Ruelfi argued that in sexual behavior, the greater the need to adapt to the practical circumstances, the greater the demand for improvisation.

As practical circumstances intrude on consciousness and impinge on action, it becomes harder and harder to ignore them. There is, in short, no choice; people must attend to them and they must attempt to adapt to them creatively if they are to prepare the sexual scene. (p. 197)

In a critique of prior writings on sexual behavior, Ruelfi further argued that social scientists often study the scripted or rule-regulated aspects of sex but ignore its improvisational aspects. As a result, this creative aspect of sex "remains uncharted and unexplored territory" (p. 191). I would argue that if we focus on the improvisational side of sex, we could derive alternative and perhaps more effective metaphors for understanding safer-sex encounters.

Safer Sex as Play

Because of its capacity to transform everyday meanings, play is the quintessential form of improvisation and creative adaptation for problematic practical circumstances. For this reason, I propose the metaphor of play for understanding safer sex.

"What is play?" A proliferation of definitions and taxonomies attest to the complexity in conceptualizing this human activity. In response to this question, Koestler (1964) attempted to clarify play's unique qualities by contrasting it with other forms of learned behavior. Koestler argued that play and humor are not to be viewed as simply forms of goal-driven behavior—but are self-reinforcing and exploratory. As such, this very human, expressive activity is emancipatory. According to Koestler, play liberates persons from the persistent endeavor to reduce drive states or to achieve specific rewards.

I use the term *play* to include a variety of communicative verbal and nonverbal exchanges that interactants find amusing (e.g., verbal play such as jokes, punning, storytelling, rhyming, metaphors, baby talk, personal idioms, role-playing; nonverbal play such as mock fighting, object play, hand games). Apart from the affective quality that these activities share, much of what is perceived as playful is accomplished by metamessages that signal "this is play" or "this is a joke" (Bateson, 1972; Goffman, 1974). These metacommunicative frames enable intimate partners to accomplish "serious relationship business" (Baxter, 1990). Although *play* and *humor* are distinctly different genres of human activity, both these terms and forms will be used interchangeably and subsumed under the term *play* in order to broaden our understanding of the improvisational and ritualized aspects for communicating about safer sex.[1]

---

[1]Although there are numerous distinctions between features of play and humor in social interaction, these distinctions are tangential to the central points of this chapter. Moreover, prior research indicates that couples use various forms of play (e.g., mock fighting) and humor (e.g., verbal tease, joking idioms) interchangeably in describing their intimate

Play and humor, however, are not without rules and structure. Most studies of play (e.g., games) emphasize its highly structured, orderly, rule-governed, and competitive qualities and ignore its more unstructured quality (Schwartzman, 1982). In her analysis of play as metaphor, Schwartzman called for interactional theories of play, where "our attention is on the ongoing communication of players as a play-event rather than on the fixed and established rules of a game" (p. 27). She proposed that text (description of the play event itself) and context (social psychological or environmental correlates of the events) cannot be treated separately, as these boundaries fuse and must be studied as a dialectical relationship.

This final point is of particular significance in the context of safer-sex discourse. The emphasis by communication researchers on intentions, strategy, and planning on the part of sexual partners serves to decontextualize the discourse. Moreover, emphasis on highly prefigurative schemas and cognitive planning suggests that sexual partners are more goal-driven and purposeful than is evident. Unlike its more strategic counterpart, negotiation, the metaphor and study of safer sex as play may shed light on the emergent, novel, and contextual features of the sexual episode.

Furthermore, this emphasis on the improvisational is crucial to understanding the new demands on erotic reality posed by the harsh threat of AIDS. This threat has inextricably linked sex with death. Undoubtedly for many newly formed sexual relationships, partners can no longer be silent about their sexual pasts nor fear to voice their concern for a sexual future. A shift from abandonment to caution now pervades the slide into passionate states. As a result, lovers are presented with the oxymoronic condition, "safer sex"—a fragile psychosocial sexual reality where innumerable tensions prevail.

The tensions apparent in this contradiction are outlined in the following section. This discussion is critical if we are to fully appreciate the significance of play and humor as mechanisms for mediating individual and relational tensions that accompany the practice of safer sex. The following underscores the primordial and preconscious behaviors that pervade sexual arousal and erotic pleasure (Givens, 1978), points to the contradictions implied by the term *safer sex,* and identifies phenomenological tensions in the practice of condom use.

SAFER SEX: AN OXYMORON

The term *safer sex* can be construed as an oxymoron (Adelman, in press) if, as some writers suggest, it is danger that actually underlies sexual ex-

---

communication (Baxter, 1990; Betcher, 1981). Subsequently, these forms are often subsumed under the more general rubric of "play." Future research may uncover relevant distinctions; however, given the paucity of work on sexual communication, broader categories can be useful in initially expanding our thinking on this topic.

citement (Stoller, 1979). In a psychoanalytical analysis of sexual excitement, Stoller described how the underlying psychic energy of arousal is
often accompanied by secrecy that serves two functions.[2] First, the
secrecy that protects us from others knowing represents the evil (i.e.,
sin) we associate with forbidden desires and our preservation of the taboo. Second, secrecy may be part of the sexual plot lines that function
to provoke or heighten arousal. This latter function appears to be an enacted but coveted form of secrecy.

This notion of secrecy is important to Stoller's major premise that
hostility (a term that covers a broad range of dangers, forbidden desires,
and repressed feelings) is the primary mechanism for sexual excitement.
His work emphasizes the oscillation between a sense of danger and a sense
of safety that gives rise to sexual arousal. He argued that in daydreams,
fantasies, and subsequently in the real world, "the delicious shudder"
is achieved by maintaining a sense of risk in the storyline. However, the
tension is achieved by building in "*safety factors* that reduce danger to
the *illusion* of danger" (p. 19). If Stoller is correct—that the subjective
experience of sexual excitement is sustained by a sense of risk or danger—
then the linguistic link between "safe" and "sex" may be interpreted as
anti-erotic.

When the idiosyncratic images that give rise to eroticism are considered, the experience of sexual excitement becomes even more complex.
The term *lovemap* is an abbreviated expression for the highly idiosyncratic image or sexual template, for the idealized sexual relationship
(Money, 1986). Similarly, the term *microdot* is used to capture the highly compressed mental data that evoke an erotic impulse (Stoller, 1979).
If danger is inherent in the templates of erotic imagination, thus giving
rise to practices that foster unprotected sex, then we need to further understand its appeal. Perhaps, rather than treating *danger* and *safety* as
polarized terms and practices, we need to understand their oscillating
qualities that could contribute to eroticizing safer sex. In short, the dialectical tension rather than the oppositional treatment of safety versus
danger may be used as an appealing invitation for its practice. For example, the term *healthy passions* in health campaigns and condom advertisements may be more appealing to erotic imagination and acts of
seduction than the more clinical term of *safer sex.*

The oxymoronic quality of safer sex also is played out in the macrolevel, schizophrenic depictions of, and prescriptions for, sexual behavior.

---

[2]Stoller (1979) is highly critical of sex research for ignoring the individual erotic experience and the psychodynamics that underlie it. In reducing sexual excitement to ana-
tomical or behavioral explanations, he argued that even "in private life, researchers know
these explanations do not fit their own histories, but curiously, in publications, the subjective experience is ignored, as if the researcher did not live in his own self" (p. 25).

Contradictions are everywhere, from regulatory practices to media imagery. We have the federal government's policy on teaching abstinence until marriage in sex education courses and the pedagogical suppression of desire (Fine, 1987). Simultaneously, we have unabashed sexual teasing 7.4 times an hour in TV soap operas, especially among unmarried couples where "in the sexually fast lane, no one ever catches a sexually transmitted disease" (Lowry & Towles, 1989, p. 81).

Cultural representations of AIDS, sex, and safer sex (e.g., messages conveyed in television programs, health campaigns, religious texts) and educational practices present an array of contradictory messages that invariably permeate the microprivate episodes of sexual encounters. As couples slide into the more climactic stages of sexual arousal they must reconcile images of sexual abandonment with cautionary tales—libido with prevention (Adelman, 1991). Practicing condom use, in some cases, conflicts with the sexual ethos of sex—threatening prevailing notions of spontaneity, naturalness, and privacy.

Psychological, relational, and physical tensions are invariably embedded in the safer-sex encounter, particularly among nonexclusive, sexually active partners. As Sontag (1989) reminded us, sex is no longer a coupling with the present, but a concern with the coupling of the past. These dialectical tensions become evident when the experience of safer sex (i.e., condom use) is contrasted with the experience of unprotected sex (Adelman, 1991), as shown in Table 4.1.

These tensions may pose serious obstacles to the practice of safer sex. Apart from specific concerns about condoms (e.g., buying, using, etc.), Miller (1990) also identified interpersonal and partner-related obstacles to using condoms. These obstacles include, for example, heat of the moment, uncomfortableness in discussing safer sex, and uncertainty about partner's reactions to using condoms. Thus, it is not only the practicalities of condom usage that pose resistance but also physical arousal, social tensions, and relational concerns that make communicating about this topic problematic.

TABLE 4.1
Tensions in Safer-Sex Encounters

Unprotected Sex	Safer Sex
spontaneity	planned
naturalness	artificial
transcendence	caution
pleasure	work
private	public
eros	logos
bios	thanatos

The relevance of play can be understood not only in terms of its contribution to relational intimacy but also in furthering our understanding in mediating the tensions and obstacles to practicing safer sex. The following section outlines the various functions of this lighter side of sexual intimacy and its implications for condom use. By identifying and labeling the functions of play we can begin to conceputalize the improvisational aspects of communication within the safer-sex context.

FUNCTIONS OF PLAY IN SAFER-SEX ENCOUNTERS

Language not only reports and stimulates lust, it forms it, and words themselves turn into erotic objects.
—Polhemus (1990, p. 262)

Several writers note the neglect of playfulness in the scholarly work on adult intimate relationships (Baxter, 1990; Bendix, 1987; Betcher, 1981; Lutz, 1982; Oring, 1984). In part, the paucity of research on this topic may reflect the nature of play itself for intimate contact. In his study of play and marital adaptation, Betcher (1981) found that playful incidents may have been forgotten by couples because of their preconscious or unconscious character. He noted that a contextual feature for play to occur is privacy. Subsequently, this subliminal and private experience of play might explain why studies of couples' sexual communication rarely detail the more playful and infantile nature of their interactions.

In the absence of this research, it is useful to consider the various functions of play and humor most relevant to sexual communication. Scholarly works on the theory and forms of play and humor derive from diverse academic disciplines. These works suggest several functions of play and humor within the safer-sex encounter, including adaptive regression, bisociation, regulating sexual arousal, constructing shared meanings, strategizing sexual invitations, coping with embarrassment, and object transformation.

Adaptive Regression

Drawing upon the studies of childhood play, psychoanalytic theory labels play in marital relationships as primarily an adaptive regression when used for "reaching the love object and modulation of ambivalence" (Betcher, 1981, p. 14). Betcher defined *intimate play* as "a spontaneous, mutual interplay in a dyadic relationship, whose content and/or style tends to be idiosyncratic and is personally elaborated by the couple" (p. 14). Play is signaled by idiosyncratic communicative acts "such as private nicknames, shared jokes and fantasies, and mock-fighting" (p. 13) and can become highly ritualized (a notion closely aligned with sexual scripts). However, Betcher noted that "the very essence of play is its creative unpredictability, and even its ritualizations have elements of improvisation" (p. 29; see Erickson, 1977).

The dialectic between danger and safety is seen in Randall's (1989) treatment of the taboo and pleasure surrounding humorous, sexual bantering. In the following excerpt, Randall spoke to the adaptive regression in adult sexual play:

> Wit, like dreams, deals with partial and disguised reappearances of forbidden impulses from the unconscious. . . . Wit or jokes present the repressed material disguised by reactivated pleasures of exhibitionism, nonsense, and wordplay. The disguises must be good enough to protect utterer and audience from feeling shame and guilt, but not so opaque as to hide completely the forbidden sexual or aggressive desire. When wit is successful, laughter represents the sudden release of energy no longer needed for repression. Pleasure is obtained from the childish play with words and momentary undoing of inhibition. The joke and the unloosening laughter provide a direct, though fleeting, communication with the unconscious. Jokes detoxify only when they succeed, that is, when they are witty or funny. The outcome is largely a quality of their disguise, which must balance protection from shame and guilt against ventilation of the forbidden wish. (pp. 29–30)

These psychoanalytic writings point to the overall function of play in regulating physical and relational tensions, often expressing, masking, or mastering anxieties (Klein, 1980). Such functions include the use of play for overcoming physical inhibition in sexual relations, for modulating aggression by introducing the absurd, for resolving crisis by reaffirmation of relational bonds, for facilitating regressive behavior to allow for risk-taking in intimate expression. Furthermore, these works indicate that play can promote social bonding in intimate relationships by signaling a shared orientation to an experience, reflecting shared values, enabling partners to recall past events, and helping to modify overly rigid personal behaviors.

Bisociation

Theories on humor and play make frequent reference to the centrality of incongruity in both the psychological and communicative accomplishment of play. An early formulation of incongruity is provided by Koestler's (1978) notion of "bisociation"—the perceiving of a situation or idea in two habitually incompatible frames of reference. Koestler described

this central feature of humor as the ability "to make the distinction between the routines of disciplined thinking within a single universe of
discourse—on a single plane, as it were—and the creative types of mental activity which always operate on more than one plane" (p. 113). He
argued that this bisociation is central to all humor. An example of these
incongruent frames is Charlie Chaplin's famous scene in the film *Modern
Times,* where he creates havoc on the factory assembly line, creating bisociation by pitting chaos against order.

Incongruity theory emphasizes the intellectual, cognitive reactions to
the unexpected, the illogical, or the inappropriate. The basic idea of incongruity theory is summarized by Morreall (1983), "We live in an orderly world, where we have come to expect certain patterns among
things, their properties, events, etc. We laugh when we experience something that doesn't fit into these patterns" (pp. 15–16). In a review of the
cognitive processes in humor, Suls (1983) argued that most humor, particularly of a verbal form, has an incongruity–resolution structure.

If humor enables consistent, but incompatible, frames of reference to
coincide, then humor in safer-sex discourse may enable sexual partners
to sustain the tension between risk and safety, the sensual and the clinical, the playful and the serious, the spontaneous and the preventative—
to reconcile seemingly incompatible states of reference in the encounter. This function of bisociation, in addition to the other functions of
play, may render "safer sex" less oxymoronic in both mind and body.

Regulating Sexual Arousal

Physiological bases for humor are also relevant for understanding play
in the context of sex. These theories propose that humor and subsequent
laughter may serve as arousal boosts or arousal jags, whereby humor
serves to increase arousal that is quickly reduced (e.g., by punchline and
resulting laughter) and presumably brings pleasure (Berlyne, 1972). This
cathartic interpretation of humor was central to Freud's contention that
laughter was the means of releasing excessive "psychic energy." Contemporary illustration of this can be found in Norman Cousins' (1979)
claims for the beneficial effects of humor in treating physical illness.
McGhee (1983) noted that laughter may help "aid in the process of return-
ing arousal [sexual] to a normal adaptive range" (p. 20), thus serving
to regulate dysfunctional levels of excitement or tension. Escalating ex-
ment prior to sexual intercourse can inhibit the discussion or practice
of condom use. Under these circumstances, the regulative function of
humor may serve to monitor and coordinate arousal for practicing safer
sex while sustaining mutual pleasure.

Constructing Shared Meanings

Fine (1983) argued that incongruity alone is not sufficient for humor, and that the social context and "idioculture," including the knowledge, beliefs, and customs of the social actors, must be taken into account. Beyond the social groupings, Fine contended that although humor is context-specific, it is formulated within the larger subterranean culture in which these groups are embedded. Similarly, Simon and Gagnon (1988) argued that sexual scripts contain elements that reflect larger cultural meanings for how to "perform" the sexual encounter. The work by Kochman (1981) on communication styles of Blacks illustrates the ways this idioculture is performed in Black culture. Kochman showed how sexual allusions and explicit sexual language are integral to the playful discourse of bantering or "rapping" between Black males and Black females. "Men rap to women in the hope of getting sex. Sometimes men rap to exercise their verbal ability; sharpen their line of wit" (p. 76).

All cultures develop norms around sexual joking and invitations to sexual relations. Sexual tease is imbued with culture-specific meanings signaling "this is sex" and "this is play." Michal-Johnson and Bowen (chapter 8, this volume) demonstrate the ways cultural meanings and practices surrounding condoms are central to understanding its resistance or utilization.

Strategizing Sexual Invitations

Sexual invitations, both in newly formed and developed relationships, tend to be ambiguous and indirect (Cupach & Metts, 1991). "Seduction, nonverbal posturing, and verbal innuendo signal sexual interests, and if responded to favorably by the partner, can become sexual initiation acts. On the other hand, if not responded to in a positive manner by the partner, they can go unacknowledged" (Cupach & Metts, 1991). These more subtle invitations enable initiating partners to assess not only mutual interest, but also to save face if overtures are rejected.

Among the numerous social functions of humor and play is the ability to communicate and assess sexual desire (Fine, 1983). Nowhere is this more evident than in testing for mutual sexual interest. Walle's (1976) ethnographic study of "pick-up" lines during closing time at bars illustrates how men move from the impersonal to the personal by telling risque jokes in order to gauge women's willingness for further contact. Thus, humor can serve as an indirect sexual invitation as well as a "test" for mutual interest in sex while minimizing the risk of rejection and loss of face.

Numerous examples in the popular press and the innovative marketing of condoms illustrate the creative combination of the safer-sex message with the sexual invitation (e.g., condoms in fortune cookies, safer-sex earrings, "condom-iments" for coffee tables, etc.). In fact, in some New York circles, wearing a safety pin has become a code that one is a practitioner of safer sex. Although the effectiveness of these combined messages in the actual practice of safer sex remains unknown, these recent developments do suggest that the semiotics of condoms are becoming a part of the playful invitation to sexual relationships.

Coping With Embarrassment

Humor may also be used in response to embarrassing situations (Edelmann, 1987; Metts & Cupach, 1989), particularly among status equals (Fink & Walker, 1977). Edelmann and Hamson (1981) found that an increase in the intimacy of the topics discussed is also accompanied by an increase in levels of embarrassment and of smiling. Humor can serve as a face-saving device to preserve a person's identity (Kane, Suls, & Tedeschi, 1977) and as a means for coping with stress (Martin & Lefcourt, 1983). Edelmann (1987) concluded that humor and laughter can change the meaning of an embarrassing situation by lessening the importance of the event and transforming the potential identity of "victim" to "co-actor."

Sexual encounters are ripe for potential embarrassment, particularly newly formed sexual relationships. Initial sexual relations are novel, unpredictable, and highly charged. In such cases, humor in safer-sex encounters may serve to sustain a desired image, to avoid losses in social approval, and to redefine a potentially embarrassing situation.

Object Transformation

Play and humor surrounding the condom itself has the capacity to transform the literal and often anti-erotic images associated with prophylactic use. Although a condom may serve as a nonverbal cue, particularly as an emblem (e.g., sign of maleness as in a condom ring in the back pocket), its presence within the sexual encounter is considered so taboo that one television commercial for condoms used the analogy of a man putting on his socks. As debates over condom commercials on television indicate, everyday meanings for condoms still connote a taboo sexual referent (Chapple & Talbot, 1989, p. 33). Given the lack of media scripts for directly discussing condom use and the awkwardness associated with its practice, humor provides a transformation of its "immodest" presence and thus depersonalizes its penile connotations.

Goffman (1974) suggested the transformational qualities of play objects when he wrote, "A plaything while in play provides some sort of ideal evidence of the manner in which a playful definition of the situation can utterly suppress the ordinary meanings of the world" (p. 43). Transformation of a play object involves a sharper differentiation between signifier and signified, wherein the object becomes a ludic symbol (objects whose practical qualities are abstracted and distorted to evoke pleasure or symbolic make believe; Piaget, 1974). "In play the emphasis changes from the question of 'What does this object do?' to 'What can I do with this object?' " (Hutt, 1976, p. 211).

As in impression management, condom management suggests that messages surrounding its presence and function can be manipulated and played with to achieve the lines of actions, or impression, most compatible with the sexual relationship. For example, a condom popping out of a drawer stuffed with hundreds of them may signal an entirely different message from one placed between the sheets or in a velvet-lined box next to the bed. In a workshop, students devised a velcro condom that would be placed behind the bedpost, thus avoiding the awkwardness of searching for one at the opportune moment. However, the idea lost its romantic appeal as the students decided that the sound of ripping velcro would be considered anti-erotic. This "prop failure" demonstrates the fragility of erotic reality (Davis, 1983) in sustaining the appropriate image of a condom user.

A scene from the film *Pretty Woman* illustrates this notion of condom management. Just prior to sex, the prostitute turns to her wealthy customer, holds up several colored condoms and says, "Pick your colors. [then smiling coyly] You look like a gold man." The message is both complimentary and direct; the playful allusion to the status of a gold credit card brings new meaning to prophylactic consumption.

In summarizing the literature on play, Glenn and Knapp (1987) wrote that "play seems to be an important act in preserving both individual and relational equilibrium. It provides an alternative to the more demanding task-oriented activity, but more importantly, the alternative may be pleasure, tension release, arousal" (p. 50). Casting these remarks in light of safer sex, play offers an alternative to the "task" or "work" associated with its practice so that the fragility of erotic reality can be sustained.

SAFER SEX: AN ILLUSTRATION
OF PLAYFUL DISCOURSE

In order to illustrate in more detail the forms and function of play for resolving the incongruities of the safer-sex encounter, I have selected excerpts of couples' safer-sex discourse from a video entitled "Safer-Sex Talk" (Adelman, Moytl, & Downs, 1988). This video includes vignettes of advanced theater students who role-played a safer-sex discussion with a sexual partner, presumably prior to engaging in sexual intercourse.[3] The following excerpts are not intended as representative samples of these couples' discourse; rather I chose only those scenes that illustrate the various ways playfulness facilitates discussion of safer sex between sexual partners. (In the scenes that follow, M = male and F = female)

Scene 1

F: Right, and I want to think about using a . . .

M: One of those.

F: I really do.

M: A . . . a raincoat (smiling up at her). Is that what you're driving at?

F: Yes, a glove.

M: (laughing) I have one of those (they kiss, then the male looking mischievously at the female). I have a whole box of them.

F: You do?

M: Pristine, unopened box. (kiss) We could use (kiss) every single one of them.

Scene 2

F: Well, actually I'm on the pill. But if you don't mind I'd like to take some precaution.

M: Double protection. Aqua Fresh (reference to a toothpaste commercial)

F: The pill doesn't protect against everything. . . . It's not like I don't trust you.

M: I understand that, but you don't have to worry, because it's not a problem.

F: Thanks.

M: I also have these condoms that a friend of mine sent me from Tijuana that have those Goodyear radial ribs on them that will drive you wild.

F: (loud laughter)

M: If you want, I don't have to drive you wild, we can have a more sedate evening.

F: No, wildness would be fine.

---

[3]In collaboration with the performers and acting director, it was decided that improvisation rather than scripted dialogues would be used to create realistic performances of sexual encounters. To emphasize variations within the scenarios the following parameters were given: (a) whether the male or female was to initiate discussion of safer sex, (b) whether the partner was to be direct or indirect in approaching this topic, (c) whether the couple was in a prearousal or postarousal sexual state, (d) whether the partner(s) were prepared or unprepared for condom usage, and (e) whether initiation of the request for safer sex resulted in compliance or resistance from the other partner. Apart from these instructions, there was no additional cuing as to whether these interactions should be serious or playful.

In both of the preceding scenes, joking about the condom serves several functions. First, it is a release from the tension raised by the female's request that the couple practice safer sex. In both cases, the female poses a justification for her request. In Scene 1 (not in text), the female notes, "I wish I had known you longer, . . ." which suggests an unfamiliarity with her partner's sexual past. In Scene 2, the female acknowledges she is on the pill but wants additional protection, which she hastens to add is not an indication that she "doesn't trust" her sexual partner. The male's response, in the form of joking about condom usage reframes the seriousness of the female's request into playful compliance by the male. The play demonstrates a form of bisociation, in particular the analogy from the toothpaste commercial that promotes the jingle of "double protection"—an absurd, but less threatening image than that posed by a sexually transmitted disease.

Playful references to the condom itself indicates a sensual transformation of its preventative connotation that displaces negative attributions about self and partner. By acknowledging the condom's object qualities as a "thing," the male displaces negative subjective meanings associated with its use or his character (e.g., prevention, questionable health). The playful reference also functions as a sexual tease. The joking response is a form of verbal foreplay that hints at the physical pleasures to come. In both excerpts, the joking response is a statement of male bravado and sexual competence. The condom is now treated as a source for sexual pleasure, thus transforming its implied everyday meaning of disease prevention into one of erotic play. Presumably, once this playful reaction is established, it would set a precedent (i.e., this is play) that would later diminish inhibitions surrounding its physical manipulation, perhaps resulting in "condom play."

In the study of other excerpts, I found that children's play forms (e.g., wordplay, hand games, horror images) were similarly used in adult sexual play—for achieving mutual agreement to engage in sexual intercourse and for introducing condom use (Adelman, 1991; see also Bell, Buerkel-Rothfuss, & Gore, 1987). In addition to providing convenient cultural scripts, these play forms may facilitate regressive, childlike behaviors that symbolize a "turning back the clock" and freedom from social constraints (Gonzales-Crussi, 1988).

CONCLUSION

Sex as an institution, sex as a general notion, sex as a problem, sex as a platitude—all this is something I find too tedious for words. Let us skip sex.
—Nabokov (1973)

Alas, even when sex carries with it the gravest danger of all—death—

it is clear that most are unlikely to join Nabokov in just "skipping" it. The advent of AIDS has revealed two rather disturbing reactions, neither of which appears receptive in ensuring responsible sexual behavior: (a) the suppression of sexuality in sex education in public schools and (b) the irresponsibility of television and film producers in addressing safer-sex behaviors while depicting sexual activity.

Rather than summarize the function of play within the sexual encounter, I conclude with a discussion of the potential for taking play seriously in addressing safer-sex practices in educational programs and depicting sexuality with heightened sensitivity in television and films.

Anti-Sex Rhetoric

In an incisive ethnographic study of sex education in public schools, Fine (1988) outlined the anti-sex rhetoric in these programs and the absence of the discourse of desire. She identified four major discourses of sexuality that reveal the ways sex education serves to control and define discourses on adolescent sexuality and to "structure silence" around adolescents' subjective experience of desire. The most prominent discourses include sexuality as violence (e.g., rape), sexuality as victimization (e.g., disease, unwanted pregnancy), and sexuality as individual morality (an emphasis on abstinence as forms of self-control and self-respect). Finally, there is the discourse of desire, "which remains a whisper inside the official work of the U.S. public schools. . . . The naming of desire, pleasure, or sexual entitlement, particularly for females, barely exists in the formal agenda of public schooling on sexuality" (pp. 31–32).

Nowhere is this anti-sex rhetoric more evident than in the new program for sex education entitled, "Sex Respect," an abstinence-based sex education curriculum that seeks to replace information about contraception and abortion with the teaching of chastity before marriage (Brotman, 1990; Watzman, 1990). Backed by the federal policy for public school sex education on "abstinence before marriage," this new curriculum even introduces the notion of "secondary virginity"—thus enabling sexually experienced females to reclaim their virgin status and renew their vows of chastity (Watzman, 1990).

Such approaches treat sex as risk-taking behavior, thus conveying a sign of recklessness and irresponsibility on the part of participants. In contrast, abstinence imbues with moral attributes those engaging in these practices. These ideological and moralistic approaches to teaching sex education do little to foster students' understanding of the psychic-erotic associations that may inhibit condom use when it is needed. Brick (1990) called for the importance of addressing sexual pleasure in teen-age sex education programs and reported on the resistance of sex educators steeped in a morally based or disease/prevention model of sex education. A focus on play and its communicative function in facilitating safer sex (specifically condom usage) could provide a framework and language in which to explore the discourse of desire, rather than its negation, in combination with learning about the practice of condom usage and abstinence.

Furthermore, sex education curriculum needs to combine cognitive, affective, and behavioral learning that encourages various ways to initiate the topic of safer sex with a potential partner. Because of the taboos and risks surrounding discussion of sex talk, conversational approaches need to consider a broad repertoire of language use (e.g., direct/indirect, serious/playful) that students perceive as plausible. Given the awkwardness in scripting or improvising sex talk, teaching methods need to consider projective techniques that can encourage nonthreatening discussion and role-plays. For example, literature, films, and television programs may be useful in getting students to identify various models of sex talk, select appropriate examples of play and humor, and possibly rewrite or even role-play a realistic or ideal scenario. Projecting personal critique and revision onto a screen or literary image may facilitate creativity, play, and open discussion that otherwise might be inhibited by lack of personal experience, peer pressure, or repercussions of self-disclosure. Regardless of the teaching method, efforts to ensure healthy sexuality must address students' subjective experience of sexual pleasure. As one student commented, "It's about time we heard the good news [in sex education]."

Media Models

Mass media offers few scripts, much less models of safer-sex practice or discourse. Television portrayals of sex scenes usually dissolve into commercial breaks, trains going into tunnels, or waves breaking onto the shore. As with educational institutions, media also structures silence around sexual discourse between partners. Apart from public service announcements on AIDS (which are restricted to late night viewing), the topic of safer sex is rarely introduced in the plot lines of prime-time television. Although research findings on media effects reveal that direct effects of media on altering viewers' behavior are questionable, there are numerous indirect effects of media in shaping viewers' responses (McQuail, 1984). For example, controversial scenes in the media often elicit public commentary about the issue at hand. Several local papers in the Chicago area commented when the television program "L.A. Law" introduced the topic of condom usage. In this show, the female partner casually tells her male lover that the condoms are in the nightstand. It was a rare moment in television history when the c-word was used in prime-time, entertainment programming.

The most dramatic illustration of a health issue promoted by mass media that gained popular acceptance was the introduction of the term *designated driver* and its subsequent practice (Winsten, 1990). Television did a great deal to dramatize this issue in prime-time programs such as "Cheers" and "The Cosby Show." Using the prestige of Harvard University, the director of the Harvard Alcohol Project, Jay Winsten, approached Hollywood producers of television programs to introduce this safety measure during prime-time viewing of entertainment shows. Within a short period, the term *designated driver* became part of American vernacular with a corresponding decrease in the number of reported drunk drivers. According to Winsten, the power of popular media far exceeded traditional health prevention campaigns in influencing public response to this critical issue.

Granted, a seductive scene between Richard Gere and Kim Basinger (pick your screen idols) performing playful talk about condom usage may not result in a dramatic change in sexual behaviors. However, their positive modeling could potentially combat the anti-erotic images surrounding condom use and reshape messages regarding unprotected sexual encounters. Ironically, the early censorship of sex on television resulted in rather playful sexual innuendos and bantering from such comics as Mae West and Groucho Marx. Hidden invitations for illicit pleasures enabled television producers to "get the message across" bypassing the censors' scissors. Perhaps, in a time of covert censorship in television, the return to play may provide a discourse in which the topic of safer sex can be introduced amidst the sexual tease and endless affairs portrayed in this media.

*   *   *

In a recent commentary in *The Journal of Sex Research,* Kayle (1990) lamented the passing of sexual passion in a decade consumed by materialism, fear appeals, paranoia, and moralizing. In short, "passion failed to make the grade in the 1980s" (p. 648). The business section of *The New York Times* detailed several projections for the 1990s; however, one trend for the next decade was described by a single word: sex. It needed no elaboration. Its starkness was evidence of its treatment in the past decade. However, unwanted pregnancy, AIDS, and other sexually transmitted diseases will remain major problems for the sexually active if education, media messages, and other cultural avenues continue to suppress the association of passion with safer-sex practices.

If our human proclivity to play is truly innate (Huizinga, 1955) perhaps it is a complementary behavior for understanding sex. If so, it is imperative to explore and affirm the function of play in sexual encounters—so as to frame sex talk in ways that can sustain healthy passions.

REFERENCES

Adelman, M. B. (1991). Play and incongruity: Framing safe-sex talk. *Health Communication, 3,* 139–155.

Adelman, M. B. (in press). Sustaining passion: Eroticism and safe-sex talk. *Archives of Sexual Behavior.*

Adelman, M. B. (Producer), Moytl, H. D. (Technical Director), Downs, D. (Acting Director). (1988). *Safe-sex Talk.* [Video]. Department of Communication Studies, Northwestern University, Evanston, IL.

Bateson, G. (1972). *Steps to an ecology of mind.* New York: Ballantine.

Baxter, L. A. (1990, November). *Intimate play in friendships and romantic relationships.* Paper presented at the annual meeting of the Speech Communication Association, Chicago.

Baxter, L. A., & Wilmont, W. W. (1985). Taboo topics in closed relationships. *Journal of Social and Personal Relationships, 2,* 253–269.

Bell, R. A., Buerkel-Rothfuss, N. L., & Gore, K. E. (1987). "Did you bring the yarmulke for the cabbage patch kid?": The idiomatic communication of young lovers. *Human Communication Research, 14,* 47–67.

Bendix, R. (1987). Marmot, memet, and marmoset: Further research on the folklore of dyads. *Western Folklore, 46,* 171–191.

Berlyne, D. E. (1972). Humor and its kin. In J. H. Goldstein & P. E. McGhee (Eds.), *The psychology of humor: Theoretical perspectives and empirical issues* (pp. 43–60). New York: Academic Press.

Betcher, R. W. (1981). Intimate play and marital adaptation. *Psychiatry, 44,* 13–33.

Brick, P. (1990, November). *Moving toward a healthy paradigm of teen sexual development.* Presentation at the annual conference for The Society for the Scientific Study of Sex, Minneapolis.

Brotman, B. (1990, May 29). Teaching students to say no to sex. *Chicago Tribune,* Tempo (Section 5), p. 1.

Burt, E. (1990–1991). Humor in erotic art. *Libido: The Journal of Sex and Sensibility, 3,* 12–17.

Chapple, S., & Talbot, D. (1989). *Burning desires: Sex in America.* New York: Doubleday.

Cousins, N. (1979). *Anatomy of an illness.* New York: Norton.

Cupach, W. R., & Metts, S. (1991). Sexuality and communication in close relationships. In K. McKinney & S. Sprecher (Eds.), *Sexuality in close relationships* (pp. 93–110). Hillsdale, NJ: Lawrence Erlbaum Associates.

Davis, M. (1983). *Smut.* Chicago: University of Chicago Press.

Edelmann, R. J. (1987). *The psychology of embarrassment.* New York: Wiley.

Edelmann, R. J., & Hampson, S. E. (1981). Embarrassment in dyadic interaction. *Social Behavior and Personality, 9,* 171–177.

Edgar, T., & Fitzpatrick, M. A. (1988). Compliance-gaining in relational interaction: When your life depends on it. *Southern Speech Communication Journal, 53,* 385–405.

Edgar, T., Freimuth, V. S., Hammond, S. L., McDonald, D. A., & Fink, E. L. (in press). Strategic sexual communication: Condom use resistance and response. *Health Communication.*

Erickson, E. (1977). *Toys and reasons: Stages in the ritualization of experience.* New York: Norton.

Fine, G. A. (1983). Sociological approaches to the study of humor. In P. E. McGhee & J. H. Goldstein (Eds.), *Handbook of humor research* (pp. 159–181). New York: Springer-Verlag.

Fine, G. A. (1987). The strains of idioculture: External threat and internal crisis on a little league baseball team. In G. A. Fine (Ed.), *Meaningful play, playful meaning* (pp. 111–128). Champaign, IL: Human Kinetics.

Fine, M. (1988). Sexuality, schooling, and adolescent females: The missing discourse of desire. *Harvard Educational Review, 58,* 29–53.

Fink, E. L., & Walker, B. A. (1977). Humorous responses to embarrassment. *Psychological Reports, 40* 475–485.

Gagnon, J. H., & Simon, W. (1973). *Sexual conduct: The social sources of human sexuality.* Chicago: Aldine.

Glenn, P. J., & Knapp, M. L. (1987). The interactive framing of play in adult conversations. *Communication Quarterly, 35,* 48–66.

Givens, D. B. (1978). The nonverbal basis of attraction: Flirtation, courtship, and seduction. *Psychiatry, 41,* 346–359.

Goffman, E. (1974). *Frame analysis.* New York: Harper & Row.

Gonzales-Crussi, R. (1988). *On the nature of things erotic.* New York: Harcourt Brace Jovanovich.

Hutt, C. (1976). Exploration and play in children. In J. S. Bruner, A. Jolly, & K. Sylva (Eds.), *Play: Its role in development and evolution* (pp. 202–215). New York: Basic Books.

Huizinga, J. (1955). *Homo ludens.* Boston: Beacon.

Kane, T. R., Suls, J., & Tedeschi, J. T. (1977). Humour as a tool of social interaction. In A. J. Chapman & H. C. Foot (Eds.), *It's a funny thing, humour* (pp. 13–16). New York: Pergamon Press.

Kayle, G. R. (1990). Whatever happened to passion? *The Journal of Sex Research, 27,* 647–649.

Klein, D. (1980). *Playfulness in marriage: A psychoanalytic perspective.* Unpublished doctoral dissertation, University of Michigan, Ann Arbor.

Kochman, T. (1981). *Black and white: Styles in conflict.* Chicago: The University of Chicago Press.

Koestler, A. (1964). *The act of creation.* New York: Dell.

Koestler, A. (1978). *Janus.* New York: Random House.

Krier, B. A. (1990, May 17). Safe sex. *Los Angeles Times* (Section E), p. 1.

Lakoff, G., & Johnson, M. (1980). *Metaphors we live by.* Chicago: University of Chicago Press.

LaPlante, M., McCormick, N., & Brannigan, G. (1980). Living the sexual script: College students' views of influence in sexual encounters. *Journal of Sex Research, 16,* 338–355.

Lowry, D. T., & Towles, D. E. (1989). Soap opera portrayals of sex, contraception, and sexually transmitted diseases. *Journal of Communication, 39,* 76–83.

Lutz, G. W. (1982). *Play, intimacy and conflict resolution: Interpersonal determinants of marital adaptation.* Unpublished doctoral dissertation, Northwestern University, Chicago.

Martin, R. A., & Lefcourt, H. M. (1983). Sense of humor as a moderator of the relation between stressors and moods. *Journal of Personality and Social Psychology, 45,* 1313–1324.

McCormick, N. B. (1979). Come-ons and put-offs: Unmarried students' strategies for having and avoiding sexual intercourse. *Psychology of Women Quarterly, 4,* 194–211.

McGhee, P. E. (1983). The role of arousal and hemispheric lateralization in humor. In P. E. McGhee & J. H. Goldstein (Eds.), *Handbook of humor research* (pp. 13–18). New York: Springer-Verlag.

McQuail, D. (1984). *Mass communication theory.* Beverly Hills: Sage.

Metts, S., & Cupach, W. R. (1989). Situational influence on the use of remedial strategies in embarrassing predicaments. *Communication Monographs, 56,* 151–162.

Metts, S., & Cupach, W. R. (1989). The role of communication in human sexuality. In K. McKinney & S. Sprecher (Eds.), *Human sexuality: The societal and interpersonal context* (pp. 139–161). Norwood, NJ: Ablex.

Miller, L. (1990, May). *Self-consciousness, interpersonal goals, and intimate negotiations: Predicting 101 obstacles to safer sex.* Paper presented at the conference on Negotiating Safer Sex, sponsored by the State of California, University-Wide Task Force on AIDS, San Diego.

Money, J. (1986). *Lovemaps.* New York: Irvington.

Morgan, G. (1986). *Images of organization.* Newbury Park, CA: Sage.

Morreall, J. (1983). *Taking laughter seriously.* Albany, NY: State University of New York.

Nabokov, V. (1973). *Strong opinions.* New York: McGraw-Hill.

Oring, E. (1984). Dyadic traditions. *Journal of Folklore Research, 21,* 19–28.

Piaget, J. (1974). Symbolic play. In J. S. Bruner, A. Jolly, & K. Sylva (Eds.), *Play: Its role in development and evolution* (pp. 555–569). New York: Basic Books.

Polhemus, R. M. (1990). *Erotic faith: Being in love from Jane Austin to D. H. Lawrence.* Chicago: University of Chicago Press.

Randall, R. S. (1989). *Freedom and taboo: Pornography and the politics of a self divided.* Berkeley: University of California Press.

Ruelfi, T. (1985). Explorations of the improvisational side of sex: Charting the future of the sociology of sex. *Archives of Sexual Behavior, 14,* 189–199.

Sarbin, T. R. (1986). The narrative as root metaphor for psychology. In T. R. Sarbin (Ed.), *Narrative psychology* (pp. 3–21). New York: Praeger.

Schwartzman, H. B. (1982). Play and metaphor. In J. W. Loy (Ed.), *The paradoxes of play* (pp. 25–33). West Point, NY: Leisure Press.

Seckman, M. A., & Couch, C. J. (1989). Jocularity, sarcasm, and relationships: An empirical study. *Journal of Contemporary Ethnography, 18,* 327–345.

Simon, W., & Gagnon, J. H. (1988). A sexual scripts approach. In J. H. Geer & W. T. O'Donohue (Eds.), *Theories of human sexuality* (pp. 363–383). New York: Plenum Press.

Sontag, S. (1989). *AIDS and its metaphors.* New York: Doubleday.

Stoller, R. J. (1979). *Sexual excitement.* New York: Simon & Schuster.

Strauss, A. (1978). *Negotiations: Varieties, contexts, processes, and social order.* San Francisco: Jossey-Bass.

Suls, K. (1983). Cognitive processes in humor appreciation. In P. E. McGhee & J. H. Goldstein (Eds.), *Handbook of humor research* (pp. 39–57). New York: Springer-Verlag.

Walle, A. (1976). Getting picked up without being put down: Jokes and the bar rush. *Journal of the Folklore Institute, 13,* 201–217.

Watzman, N. (1990, July/August). When sex ed becomes chastity class. *Utne Reader,* 92–97.

Winsten, J. A. (1990, October). *The Harvard Alcohol Project: A demonstration project to promote the use of the "Designated Driver."* Presented at the annual conference for the Association for Consumer Research, New York.

CHAPTER FIVE

Theoretical Foundations of AIDS Media Campaigns

Vicki S. Freimuth
University of Maryland

Until a cure or vaccine is found, prevention is the most important weapon against the AIDS epidemic. The mass media, especially television, have always been attractive channels for prevention messages because they have the potential of quickly and inexpensively disseminating information to millions of people. Chapter 7 by Salmon and Kroger describes "America Responds to AIDS," the largest of these American AIDS media campaigns, and chapter 6 by Marková and Power describes the British use of mass media to encourage AIDS prevention.

Evidence exists that these campaigns are reaching the public. The Centers for Disease Control, for example, estimates its AIDS messages received $18 million in free time and space in 1988 ("A misfire in the AIDS fight," 1988). In addition, a National Center for Health Statistics survey conducted in August 1988 found that 84% of all adults in the United States reported having seen AIDS public service announcements (PSAs) on television (Centers for Disease Control, 1988). Wallack (1990) reported national survey findings that television was the most frequently mentioned source of AIDS information, cited more than twice as often as newspapers and 25 times as often as physicians.

Increased awareness certainly has followed from this exposure. For several years now, surveys consistently have documented that the American public are aware of AIDS and know the basic ways it is transmitted although a few still harbor some misconceptions. Even behavioral change has been identified among homosexuals and IV drug users although not among adolescent heterosexuals (Becker & Joseph, 1988).

Yet mass media campaigns are not a panacea for AIDS prevention. Most of these campaigns rely on televised PSAs as their primary channels. PSAs have some serious limitations. Because the air time is donated rather than purchased, PSAs often are aired at times when few members of the target audience are watching. Moreover, PSAs must be very brief messages, usually no more than 30 seconds. PSAs also have to compete with slickly produced commercial advertisements, both for air time and audience attention.

In health communication campaigns, it is not uncommon for less than 10% of the target audience to report seeing any of the campaign messages. A number of processes work to consistently narrow the audience for these campaigns. Hammond, Freimuth, and Morrison (1987) presented a funnel model of the gatekeeping process showing how a PSA with a potential of reaching more than 170 million Americans may be broadcast to only 14% of homes with televisions and achieve a response in fewer than 1% of the potential viewers. Even though a PSA is distributed to every television station in the country, only a small percentage of these stations actually air the spot. The funnel narrows even further when the PSA reaches the audience, who selectively expose themselves to messages, avoiding exposure to messages in which they have no interest.

The limitations of PSA campaigns are compounded when the subject is AIDS. AIDS requires discussing sensitive issues such as explicit sexuality and death and dying. The target audiences for many AIDS prevention messages are small, stigmatized groups such as homosexuals or IV drug users, audiences out of the mainstream of normal television programming. Winett, Altman, and King (1990) identified additional obstacles in designing effective AIDS campaigns:

1. the problems involved in presenting explicit messages on network television or in public places
2. the focus on changing private behaviors that cannot be observed and sometimes are illegal
3. the importance of altering specific behaviors since HIV can spread through only one contact
4. the need to prevent behavioral lapses and relapses since they can be fatal. (p. 92)

A content analysis of over 100 AIDS PSAs (Freimuth, Hammond, Edgar, & Monahan, 1990) suggested that the media may be avoiding these challenges by developing messages for general audiences, recommending only the most noncontroversial preventive behaviors (e.g., information seeking), and failing to address the barriers to behavior change.

Certainly, media campaigns fall squarely within the purview of communication scholars. The central question guiding this chapter was what theoretical guidance can communication scholars offer planners of AIDS media campaigns? First, I offer a working definition of the term *campaign,* explaining what is included and excluded. Second, I review typologies of theories useful for health communication campaigns and describe applications of selected theories to AIDS media campaigns. Finally, I conclude the chapter with a discussion of the insights gained from applying theories to AIDS campaigns.

DEFINITIONS OF MEDIA CAMPAIGNS

Campaigns are "organized attempts to influence another's beliefs about, attitudes toward, and/or behaviors with respect to some object (e.g., product, issue, person, etc.) through the use of mass media or other communication channels" (Devine & Hirt, 1989, p. 230).

The following four elements are common to campaigns:

1. Campaigns are purposeful and seek to influence individuals.
2. Campaigns are aimed at large audiences.
3. Campaigns are conducted for specific periods of time.
4. Campaigns include an organized set of communication activities (Rogers & Storey, 1987).

I am excluding from this chapter any discussion of brief educational interventions limited to small audiences such as safe sex workshops and AIDS educational videotapes.

Even though campaigns may represent one of the most applied areas of communication research, they draw heavily on theories to improve their effectiveness. Salmon (1989) distinguished between theory of campaigns and theory for campaigns. Theories of campaigns concern the social context in which campaigns occur and are addressed in chapter 6 by Marková and Power. This chapter focuses on theory for campaigns, examining those theories that can guide the development of messages and the choice of channels in AIDS campaigns.

TYPOLOGIES OF THEORIES USED IN CAMPAIGNS

Almost any theory explaining human behavior could be relevant to an AIDS media campaign, so identifying and organizing them can be a daunting task. Winett et al. (1990) argued convincingly that campaign design and implementation is an interdisciplinary effort, requiring a multidisciplinary team of professionals. The disciplines usually represented include psychology, communication, public health, health education, marketing, sociology, and anthropology. Several researchers have developed typologies of theories potentially applicable to campaigns. In the following sections, I describe four of these typologies, ranging from the simpler to the more complex.

Source, Message, Channel Typology

Perloff and Pettey (1991), from the communication discipline, organized theories in terms of the basic "who (source) says what (message) through which modality (channel)" model of communication. For source factors, they advised that AIDS campaigns are more effective if they use spokespersons who are perceived as credible by the target audience. For campaigns targeted at IV drug users they recommended that "insiders" be used, perhaps IV drug users who formerly shared needles but now use bleach to clean needles or IV drug users who have come in for treatment rather than celebrities or authority figures.

They singled out fear as the message factor most relevant for AIDS campaigns. For campaigns targeted to IV drug users, they recommended that fear messages should contain four components: (a) information about the magnitude of the problem, (b) high probability that the negative consequences will occur if behaviors are not changed, (c) an action plan to show how the consequences can be reversed, and (d) assurance that the person is fully capable of undertaking these behaviors (self-efficacy).

In discussing channel factors, they pointed out the importance of supplementing mass media with interpersonal channels. For IV drug users, they recommended using outreach workers to disseminate the messages in target messages.

Message-Based and Behavioral-Based Typology

Psychologists Devine and Hurt (1989) classified psychological theories applied in campaigns into message-based and behavioral-based, suggesting that the critical distinction between them is the source of the initial information that provides the basis for the attitude (i.e., either a message from a communicator or the recipient's own experience). In message-based theories, communications are constructed to convey information about the attitude object with the expectation that the arguments presented will elicit positive attitudes in the audience that will, in turn, lead to positive behaviors. Examples given of these theories are McGuire's (1989) information-processing model, Greenwald's (1968) cognitive response theory, and Petty and Cacioppo's (1986) Elaboration-Likelihood Model. In contrast, the behavioral-based theories assume that behavior precedes attitude change (i.e., getting the audience to perform the recommended behavior leads to attitude change). Examples of these theories include social-learning theory (Bandura, 1969, 1977), dissonance theory (Festinger, 1957), and operant conditioning (Skinner, 1957).

Devine and Hirt (1989) offered campaign planners guidance for selecting the appropriate class of theories to use. They recommended message-based theories when mass media are available and affordable, interpersonal communication is less feasible, the topic permits a compelling and understandable message, the audience is somewhat familiar with the issues, and the goal is to stimulate repeated behaviors. Behavioral-based theories, they argued, are more suitable when interpersonal channels are more available than mass media ones, the audience is less familiar with the issues, and the goal is to produce one-time behaviors and/or repeated behaviors.

Directive and Dynamic Typology

McGuire (1989), another psychologist, presented an overlapping but somewhat different conceptual scheme to organize psychological theories useful to campaign planners. He offered two categories: directive and dynamic theories. Directive theories describe how a person processes the social influence advocated in public communication campaigns, whereas dynamic theories explain the forces that drive the person to engage in the processing.

McGuire offered a comprehensive information-processing model in the form of an input/output matrix as the example of a directive theory. The output or dependent variables are response steps mediating persuasion and include exposure, attending, comprehending, yielding, and retaining. The independent communication variables include source, message, channel, receiver, and destination characteristics. His input/output matrix provides a framework for organizing much of the research conducted on campaigns. Flay and Burton (1990) labeled this order of effects model as the learning hierarchy (i.e., knowledge is changed first, then attitudes, and finally, behaviors). They suggested that this sequence is appropriate for salient issues in which the target audience is highly involved and where alternative choices are very different, conditions consistent with high-risk, highly motivated audiences in AIDS campaigns. Rogers and Story (1987) included this hierarchical model of communication effects with such others as Ray's (1973) cognitive/affective/conative hierarchy, Fishbein and Ajzen's (1975) belief/attitude/intention/behavior model, and the knowledge/persuasion/decision/confirmation stages of the innovation-decision process described by Rogers (1983).

Devine and Hurt (1989) criticized these hierarchical models for their assumption that these response stages occur in a fixed sequence and failure to produce one stage stops the persuasion process. They also argued that these models do not address why a stage does or does not occur (e.g., what is the process that results in one yielding to a message?).

Flay and Burton (1990) identified two alternative orders of effects models: the low-involvement hierarchy and the dissonance-attribution hierarchy. The low-involvement hierarchy is appropriate when people are not involved in the issue and there are minimal differences between alternatives. Much product advertising falls into this category but it is less appropriate for AIDS campaigns. The third order of effects model, the dissonance-attribution hierarchy, describes those situations when people are involved in an issue where the alternatives are quite similar, they may try something, decide they like it, and then selectively attend to information that supports their decision. This model may explain the effects of those AIDS campaigns that encourage empathy toward persons with AIDS or donation of money or time to AIDS related causes.

McGuire's second category of psychological theories, the dynamic theories, focuses on human motivation and is organized into four families based on forces that initiate human action, whether stability or growth, and forces that have to do with end states that terminate action, cognitive or affective. This two-by-two matrix creates four families of theories, the cognitive stability theories (e.g., consistency), the cognitive growth theories (e.g., autonomy), the affective stability theories (e.g., ego-defensive), and the affective growth theories (e.g., social learning).

Behavioral Systems Typology

The most ambitious typology, developed by Winett et al. (1990), crosses disciplinary lines and includes the following theories: social cognitive theory, communication theory, process of change schema, community organization, diffusion of innovation, public health approach, developmental/ecological perspective, social marketing, and behavioral systems. Table 5.1 outlines the significance and an application example for each of these theories. These authors attempted to integrate all of these theories into a behavioral systems framework for program conceptualization, design, implementation, and evaluation. They applied this framework to the design of a media and community campaign for AIDS prevention with adolescents. Table 5.2 presents an outline of the campaign steps, concepts, principles, procedure, and methods.

The objective of the campaign is to get heterosexuals to use condoms

TABLE 5.1

Conceptual Foundations for Media Campaigns

Theory/Framework/ Perspective	Significance	Example of an Application
Social cognitive theory	Principles and strategies of individual behavior change	Use of modeling principles in media
Communication theory	Principles for information processing, delivery system design	Organize information for retention enhancement
Process of change schema	Ordering of principles and strategies for stages of behavior change	Successive change steps in a campaign to change individual behavior
Community organization	Principles and strategies for change in community systems	Organization of community resources to facilitate a media campaign
Diffusion of innovation	Principles and strategies for adoption and spread of innovations	Augment a media campaign with an interpersonal component
Public health approach	Principles and strategies for preventive interventions	Combining "passive" and "active" prevention methods in one campaign
Developmental/Ecological perspective	Focus on critical periods, roles, and settings	Target people at critical transition points in life in particular settings
Social marketing	Overarching elements of a campaign	Product design, price, promotion, place, and positioning
Behavioral systems	Integration and ordering of principles and strategies	Optimize design, community aspects, delivery, and evaluation of a campaign

Note: From Winett et al. (1990. Copyright © 1990, Pergamon Press)

TABLE 5.2

Outline of a Media and Community Campaign for AIDS Prevention in Adolescents

Steps	Concepts, Principles, Procedures, Methods
Problem Definition	Concepts/Principles
Individual—beliefs, knowledge, particular behavior	Social cognitive—modeling
Interpersonal—peer, group norms, expectations	Communication—Specific prescriptions
Organizational/Community—availability issues	Community organization acceptability/parental
Institutional/Societal—legal constraints	Process of change—series of steps from initial to long-term change
Multilevel Analysis	Diffusion—respected peers
Overcome individual and interpersonal barriers	Developmental/Ecological—specific age group; delivery in proper settings
Provide in school or community availability plus counseling	Social marketing—tailoring to different locations
Peer Facilitators	
Multidimensional evaluation (e.g., beliefs, reported behaviors, sales, distribution, morbidity, social indicators)	
Intervention Design	Procedures
PSA series within MTV following process of change schema	Modeling via PSA series and valued peers
Specific scenes, characters, and prescriptions based on age and location	Prescriptive—step-by-step approach
	Benefits for participating agencies
	Specifically design and target different PSAs for different ages and localities

Manuals and facilitator (health education) for school and/or
community to increase condom availability, parent education,
and counseling
Specific goals for knowledge, behavior change, condom distribution,
pregnancy STD incidence
Specific measure for each goal
Formative research initial pilot testing

Intervention Implementation
Pilot testing
Optimal population and location
Integrity (e.g., reach of PSAs, ease of availability)
Continual data feedback and refinements

Evaluation
Checks for contaminations between media markets
Outcomes on each measure compared to goals and control commu-
nities
Test for hypothesized process of change
Impacts across communities
Plan of replication series
Cost per unit of change

Models for adoption
Active prevention—school and/or community-based
procedure

Methods
True experiment—random assignment of communities
(Media markets)
Multiple measure for major goals
Process of change
Cost figures

Note: From Winett et al. (1990. Copyright © 1990, Pergamon Press)

during intercourse. Winett et al. (1990) did caution planners to set realistic goals such as a 25% decrease in reports of unprotected sexual behavior and a 20% increase in sales and distribution of condoms. The centerpiece of the campaign is a series of explicit PSAs on Music Television (MTV) along with the availability of condoms in schools and community settings. Extensive formative and developmental research is conducted as a basis for designing the PSA's content. A series of PSAs follows the process of change schema with the first ones focusing on outcome expectancies and increasing self-efficacy, later ones on skill building, and final ones emphasizing maintenance of the behaviors.

These typologies differ in respect to their disciplinary origin, their inclusiveness, and their complexity. Although AIDS campaign planners may find these typologies useful in identifying and organizing relevant theories, further examples are necessary to demonstrate how AIDS media campaigns have applied specific theories to message design or program planning. In the next section, I present five specific theories that have been applied in AIDS media campaigns. The first two theories, the Health Belief Model (HBM) and cognitive-social learning theory, frequently are used to guide the choice of persuasive appeal or strategy. The latter three theories—diffusion of innovations, social marketing, and media advocacy—are more useful in the campaign planning process.

THEORY APPLICATION

The Health Belief Model

This model was developed in the 1950s by individuals in the Public Health Service to explain public participation in screening programs. The model suggests that readiness to engage in a health behavior follows from a perceived threat of disease, coming from an individual's perception of his or her susceptibility to the disease and its potential severity (Becker, (1974). The cue for action is a triggering device stimulated by a private perception or by communication from the media or other people. Behavior is evaluated from an estimate of the potential benefits of engaging in the recommended health behavior to reduce susceptibility or severity. The benefits are then weighed against perceptions of physical, psychological, financial, and other costs or barriers inherent in the recommended health behavior. Demographic, social, structural, and personality factors are included in the model because they are believed to indirectly influence behavior.

Even though the HBM has been used to explain risk-taking behavior related to HIV infection and to predict change in HIV-preventive behaviors (Catania, Kegeles, & Coates, 1990; Emmons et al., 1986; McKusick, Horstman, & Coates, 1985), the results have been disappointing. Brown, DiClemente, and Reynolds (1991) identified the following limitations of the HBM for HIV prevention for adolescents: difficulty accounting for change of habitual behaviors, relative exclusion of emotional reactions and peer-group influence, and lack of maturational constructs. In general, the HBM is a rational-cognitive model and assumes a "rational" decision maker. Most adolescents, and many adults, do not seem to approach the AIDS issue from such a logical perspective but seem quite capable of discounting risks and optimistically perceiving themselves as invulnerable to harm.

Cognitive-Social Learning Theory

Campaign planners also have frequently turned to cognitive-social learning theory (Bandura, 1986) to guide AIDS prevention efforts. This theory recognizes the reciprocity among cognitive, behavioral, environmental, and physiological/affective influences. A person's behavior, then, depends on the interactive effects of these influences. Two specific principles from this theory that have received considerable application in AIDS campaigns include modeling and self-efficacy.

Modeling is a strategy that encourages the imitation of the behavior of another well-respected person. This principle acknowledges that people learn from a variety of experiences, often vicariously by observing the actions of others.

Modeling was the strategy apparently used in an AIDS PSA targeted toward young adolescents in a Seattle campaign (Freimuth et al., 1990). As a teen-age couple dances at a party, the audience hears their internal thoughts and dialogue:

Boy (thinking to self): I wonder if she'd go out to the car with me. I meant to buy a rubber, but it's not easy and it can be embarrassing. Maybe she's on the pill.

Girl (thinking to self): I want to be closer to him but I don't want to get pregnant, and I suppose I should worry about AIDS.

Boy (talking aloud): Let's go back to the car.

Voice-over: Think before you go back to the car.

Girl (talking aloud): Are you protected?

Voice-over: Learn to talk to each other. Deciding to have sex is a serious matter.

The second principle, perceived self-efficacy, concerns people's judgment about their own ability to enact recommended behaviors. Some AIDS campaigns have taught negotiation of safe sex skills in an attempt to increase self-efficacy regarding condom use. Flora and Thoresen (1988) suggested that AIDS campaigns include messages that teach people to "inoculate" themselves against social pressures in real life. Yet Freimuth et al.'s (1990) analysis of AIDS PSAs revealed that only a few (7%) of the messages portrayed a real-life situation and an equally small number discussed the difficulties in enacting the recommended behaviors. Of those PSAs that showed poor interpersonal communication as a barrier to successful practice of safe sex, two did not address the issue beyond a veto on sexual intercourse. For example, one produced in New York City opens with a young heterosexual couple kissing. After she places a condom in his hand, he refuses to use it. Her response is to say "forget it" and walk away. One could question whether this spot increases self-efficacy. Instead, by resolving the conflict with a veto on sexual intercourse, it may negatively reinforce the recommended behavior.

Flora and Thoresen (1988) provided an excellent example of translating cognitive-social learning theory into practice. They recommended a series of steps to follow in developing AIDS prevention programs for young adolescents. The first step was to conduct a cognitive-behavioral analysis of the antecedents, concomitant behaviors, and immediate consequences of sexual activity of adolescents. Such information should yield a social learning history to facilitate understanding of the sexual experience for these young people. The second step was to use this information to (a) identify high-risk situations, (b) identify pressures to engage in sex, (c) create role-play situations that are realistic to teen-agers, (d) capture the words, phrases, and syntax of teen language, and (e) identify gender, ethnic, and racial similarities and differences. The third and final step Flora and Thoresen outlined was to structure these formative data according to cognitive social learning theory principles using creative implementation strategies such as peer models and role-playing. Environmental and social support for the teens could come from education of parents, teachers, and other significant adults.

Diffusion of Innovations

Diffusion of innovations is the process of communicating about new ideas through channels over time among the members of a particular social system (Rogers, 1983). The most widely quoted principle from this theory is that the mass media are most useful for stimulating awareness of a new idea and communicating information about it. When trying to persuade an audience to adopt a new or behavior, interpersonal channels are more effective. This principle has frequently guided AIDS campaigns to rely on mass media (often PSAs) to achieve awareness and dissemination of knowledge (e.g., see Salmon & Kroger, chapter 7, this volume) and on small-group interventions for persuasion.

A second principle from diffusion of innovations theory that has received wide application in AIDS campaigns is the use of opinion leaders. Opinion leaders are those individuals who are similar to the target audience but are able to influence others' attitudes or behaviors informally (Rogers, 1983). Often in AIDS campaigns, community-based organizations are used as opinion leaders to disseminate messages to their constituencies. In addition, intravenous drug users have been reached in many campaigns by enlisting the help of former IV drug users as opinion leaders (Perloff & Pettey, 1991).

Some of the criticisms advanced against this theory are especially relevant for its application in AIDS campaigns. Diffusion of innovations has been criticized for being too linear, for having a pro-innovation bias, and for widening the gaps between the "information haves" and "have-nots" in a social system. This gap has certainly been observed in AIDS awareness and knowledge. The more highly educated segments of society consistently demonstrate greater awareness and more indepth knowledge of AIDS than do the poor and minority groups (Mays & Cochran, 1988).

Social Marketing

The marketing discipline has contributed an approach quite similar to diffusion of innovations—social marketing. This field was born in 1952, when Wiebe asked, "Why can't you sell brotherhood like you sell soap?" (Solomon, 1989). As the concept of marketing as an exchange process was expanded beyond commercial transaction, the field of social marketing developed. This new field was defined as:

> the design, implementation, and control of programs seeking to increase the acceptability of a social idea or practice in a target group(s). It utilizes concepts of market segmentation, consumer research, concept development, communication, facilitation, incentives, and exchange theory to maximize target group response. (Kotler, 1984, p. 24)

Perhaps the best known set of concepts from social marketing is the four Ps: product, price, place, and promotion. The product in social marketing, unlike commercial marketing, is not necessarily a physical entity. It can consist only of ideas, practices, or services. For AIDS campaigns, the product could be searching for more information about the disease, getting an HIV test, demonstrating empathy toward HIV positive individuals, or using condoms. The price of a product or service involves more than the monetary cost. It may include time, pain, embarrassment, or anxiety associated with "purchasing." Place in social marketing refers to distribution channels used to make the product or service available to the target audience. AIDS campaigns on college campuses, for example, frequently use the health center or the dormitory as the place to distribute free condoms. The fourth "P" is promotion and includes all those activities that make the consumer aware of the product or service and encourage them to develop appropriate attitudes toward it and ultimately to enact desired behaviors. In the AIDS campaigns, the mass-mediated messages such as PSAs, posters, and brochures would be examples of promotion.

Social marketing also has critics such as Wallack (1990) who identified several limitations. This theory is often considered ethically suspect and manipulative, perhaps because of its close association with the advertising and marketing of commercial products. Social marketing also has been criticized for promoting single solutions to complex health problems (e.g., use condoms to stop AIDS) and not addressing the social conditions that cause and sustain disease.

The social marketing approach has been adapted by the U.S. Public Health Service into the Health Communication Process, a six-stage circular process in which feedback is solicited continuously from the consumers (U.S. Department of Health and Human Services, 1989). Figure 5.1 shows this six-stage process model. Stage 1, the planning and strategy selection phase, provides the foundation for the entire process. During this stage, the planners identify and analyze existing information about the issue and potential target audiences, they decide if any additional research is necessary, what specific change is desired, what the measurable objectives are, how progress can be measured, and draft the communication strategies.

In Stage 2, the planners select channels and materials for the campaign. They may assess existing materials to determine whether they can be used, decide on appropriate channels to reach the target audiences, and choose the formats for the messages (e.g., PSAs, brochures, comic books).

The campaign planners actually develop and pretest materials during Stage 3. Audience feedback is critical at this stage of the process. Draft materials are pretested with members of the target audiences to assess the materials' attention-getting value, comprehensibility, relevance, and persuasiveness. Materials are usually revised following this feedback. Planners also develop promotion and distribution systems during this stage.

The fully developed campaign is introduced to the target audience during Stage 4, the implementation phase. During this phase, the campaign is continuously monitored and revised, if necessary, to assure that the

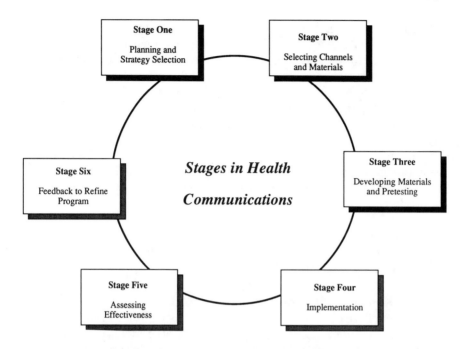

FIG. 5.1.   Stages in health communication. (From Department of Health and Human Services, 1989).

messages are making it through the channels and reaching and impacting the target audiences.

Effectiveness of the campaign is assessed during the fifth stage using the measurable objectives formulated during Stage 1. In addition to measuring whether the objectives were met, the planners also note unintended effects and evaluate the planning process itself.

Finally, in Stage 6, all this information gathered about the target audiences, the messages, the channels, and the campaign's effectiveness is fed back into the process to inform the next planning cycle. This model is an excellent example of how a more abstract theory such as social marketing is translated into a pragmatic set of guidelines for campaign planners.

Media Advocacy

Both diffusion of innovations and social marketing use the media to promote change in individual health behaviors. Media advocacy is a new approach that is a fundamentally different use of the media for public health purposes (Wallack, 1990). It targets policy rather than individual change and participates aggressively in the news arena rather than relying on public service. Media advocacy stimulates media coverage in order to reframe public debate to increase support for more effective policies. The goal of media advocacy is to empower the public to participate more fully in defining the social and political environment in which decisions affecting health are made. ACT-UP is the activist group that has used media advocacy to effect change in AIDS public policies. This activist group tries to manipulate the media to gain control over the apparatus by which the disease is interpreted to the public. They have used such techniques as unplugging microphones, jamming fax machines, chaining themselves to news desks, hurling themselves in front of cameras, and heckling speakers (Harris, 1991).

INSIGHTS GAINED FROM APPLYING THEORIES TO AIDS CAMPAIGNS

The AIDS epidemic confronts the public health community with a deadly disease where their only available weapon is prevention through public education and persuasion. The pressure on AIDS media campaigns has been enormous. Many principles well-established in other health campaigns had to be relearned by AIDS policymakers. Because of the sensitive subject matter surrounding AIDS and the stigmatized target audiences, health communicators have faced some new challenges. In the following section, I highlight some of the insights gained from applying theories from a variety of disciplines to AIDS media campaigns. Some of these insights are not new but have received considerable attention because of the AIDS epidemic.

Knowledge is a Necessary but not Sufficient Condition for Behavior Change. Health communicators discovered this principle long ago as illustrated in smoking cessation efforts. Most smokers know that their behavior is harmful but many have not stopped. The early AIDS campaigns appeared to assume that information was all that was needed and once the public understood how to stop AIDS, they would act rationally and adopt recommended behaviors. The lack of correlation between knowledge and behavior change eventually convinced AIDS policymakers otherwise. Although the theories under discussion can offer guidance for motivating behavior change, media campaigns have traditionally been used to stimulate awareness, leaving the subsequent steps of the behavior-change process to more interpersonal sources. Yet, a few media campaigns have included motivational messages. Over time, the research generated about AIDS media campaigns may change the conventional wisdom that mass media can only stimulate awareness but have little impact on actual behavior.

The American Public is not a Monolith but a Group of Highly Diverse Audiences. Hyman and Sheatsley (1947) first identified this principle in their article, "Some Reasons Why Information Campaigns Fail" and advocated targeting messages to specific segments of the public. Yet most of the earliest AIDS media campaigns and many current ones still target the general public without acknowledging the differences among such segments as homosexuals, bisexuals, women, adolescent heterosexuals, IV drug users, and minority groups. Not only are the segments quite diverse but the process each one undergoes in changing behavior also may be different. Mays and Cochran (1988) argued eloquently for recommending different persuasive strategies for women of color because they operate within different cultural norms than their White, middle-class sisters. Segmentation of audiences is a fundamental part of social marketing, one of the process theories described earlier, but as Michal-Johnson and Bowen (chapter 8) explain, most of the theories used in developing campaign strategies do not include culture as a central concept. The AIDS epidemic as well as the increasing diversity in the population will most likely force the integration of culture into many of these models.

Maintaining Behavior Change is a Different Challenge Than Initiating Behavior Change. A few recommended health behavior changes require only a one-time enactment, others demand repeated but infrequent action (e.g., having a Pap test once a year), and some necessitate continuous maintenance such as eating low fat foods. AIDS prevention is one that requires frequent practice of recommended behaviors (e.g., using a condom), but the uniqueness of AIDS prevention is that recidivism could be fatal. Hence, maintenance of behavior change takes on an urgency seldom seen in previous campaigns. Many of the theories being applied focus only on initiating behavior change and do not offer any guidance for maintaining that change over time.

Audiences Traditionally Labeled "Hard-to-Reach" Cannot be Ignored. Historically, the poor and minorities have suffered disproportionally from most diseases. In the past, their suffering did not always threaten the majority population or drain the system of as many resources as does AIDS. Consequently, these disadvantaged groups cannot be ignored and have become the primary target audiences for many HIV/AIDS prevention campaigns. Campaign planners who usually are from a different social class and ethnic group from their target audiences are forced to recognize their limited understanding and seek new ways to learn about and reach these audiences. In the process, assumptions are being shattered. For example, as IV drug users were first targeted for AIDS prevention messages, planners assumed they were self-destructive or, at least, apathetic. Evaluations of these campaigns demonstrated that change was occurring and these populations wanted to prevent HIV infection (Des Jarlais & Friedman, 1988).

The Norms of Media Gatekeepers, the Public, and Policymakers can be Changed Slowly. Early public discussions about HIV/AIDS used euphemisms such as "bodily fluids" and other vague terms. Gradually, more explicit language was accepted and the word "condom" became commonplace. In Seattle, a television station produced a PSA that featured two homosexuals discussing AIDS. Models of the gatekeeping process may need to be altered to reflect the effect of public pressure on the gatekeepers' traditional roles.

The Dichotomy Between Interpersonal and Mass Communication is a False One, Detrimental to Effective AIDS Media Campaigns. AIDS campaigns should not rely on the mass media alone to produce behavior change. Studies of the effects of mass media campaigns have moved over the past several decades from simplistic descriptions of a "hypodermic needle" effect, a direct and universal response to the media, to the two-step flow model, where messages flow from the media to opinion leaders who then disseminate them to others, to, more recently, the multistep flow model, where messages can reach audiences directly or through many layers of interpersonal contacts (Rogers, 1983). AIDS campaigns to reach IV drug users frequently implement this multistep flow by supplementing mass media messages with outreach workers, who engage members of the target audience in one-on-one dialogues about prevention.

CONCLUSION

These six principles demonstrate the impact that the HIV/AIDS epidemic has had on health communication campaigns. The content of the messages has expanded the boundaries of community acceptability. Audiences formerly ignored by programmers and advertisers have become the targets of AIDS campaigns. The channel selection has had to accommodate small, stigmatized groups without offending the larger, spill-over audiences. Because of the urgency of the HIV/AIDS epidemic, the theories traditionally applied to health communication campaigns have been subjected to intense scrutiny. Some, such as the Health Belief Model, have not held up very successfully; others, such as cognitive-social learning, seem more promising.

Earlier, I indicated that the central question of the chapter was what theoretical guidance we could offer to campaign planners. The typologies of theories potentially applicable to these campaigns as well as the examples of applications of specific theories demonstrate that considerable guidance is available and currently being used. But, perhaps, the most intriguing question is: What impact will these AIDS applications have on the development of our theories? I have noted that many of the theories do not incorporate culture as a central construct, do not address maintenance of behaviors, and make assumptions about human behavior that may be fallacious (e.g., rational decision making). Applying our theories to prevent a real and devastating disease may stimulate their improvement.

REFERENCES

A misfire in the AIDS fight. (1988, October 24). *Advertising Age,* p. 16.

Bandura, A. (1969). *Principles of behavioral modification.* New York: Holt, Reinhart & Winston.

Bandura, A. (1977). *Social learning theory.* Englewood Cliffs, NJ: Prentice-Hall.

Bandura, A. (1986). *Social foundations of thought and action: A social cognitive theory.* Englewood Cliffs, NJ: Prentice-Hall.

Becker, M. H. (Ed.). (1974). *The health belief model and personal health behavior.* Thorofare, NJ: Charles B. Slack.

Becker, M. H., & Joseph, J. G. (1988). AIDS behavioral change to reduce risk: A review. *American Journal of Public Health, 78,* 394–410.

Brown, L. K., DiClemente, R. J., & Reynolds, L. A. (1991). HIV prevention for adolescents: Utility of the health belief model. *AIDS Education and Prevention, 3,* 50–57.

Catania, J. A., Kegeles, S. M., & Coates, T. J. (1990). Towards an understanding of risk behavior: An AIDS risk reduction model. *Health Education Quarterly, 17,* 53–72.

Centers for Disease Control. (1988, August). *AIDS knowledge and attitudes* (DHHS Publication No. PHS 89-1250). Hyattsville, MD: National Center for Health Statistics.

Des Jarlais, D. C., & Friedman, S. R. (1988). The psychology of preventing AIDS among intravenous drug users: A social learning conceptualization. *American Psychologist, 43*(11), 865–870.

Devine, P. G., & Hirt, E. R. (1989). Message strategies for information campaigns: A social psychological analysis. In C. T. Salmon (Ed.), *Information campaigns: Balancing social values and social change* (pp. 229–258). Newbury Park, CA: Sage.

Emmons, C. A., Joseph, J. G., Kessler, R. C., Wortman, C. B., Montgomery, S. B., & Ostrow, D. G. (1986). Psychosocial predictors of reported behavior change in homosexual men at risk for AIDS. *Health Education Quarterly, 13,* 331–345.

Festinger, L. A. (1957). *A theory of cognitive dissonance.* Evanston, IL: Row Peterson.

Fishbein, M., & Ajzen, I. (1975). *Belief, attitude, intention and behavior: An introduction to theory and research.* Reading, MA: Addison-Wesley.

Flay, B. R., & Burton, D. (1990). Effective mass communication strategies for health campaigns. In C. Atkin & L. Wallack (Eds.), *Mass communication and public health* (pp. 129–146). Newbury Park, CA: Sage.

Flora, J. A., & Thoresen, C. E. (1988). Reducing the risk of AIDS in adolescents. *American Psychologist, 43,* 965–970.

Freimuth, V. S., Hammond, S. L., Edgar, T., & Monahan, J. L. (1990). Reaching those at risk: A content-analytic study of AIDS PSAs. *Communication Research, 17*(6), 775–791.

Greenwald, A. (1968). Cognitive learning, cognitive response to persuasion and attitude change. In A. Greenwald, T. Brock, & T. Ostrom (Eds.), *Psychological foundations of attitudes* (pp. 361–388). New York: Academic Press.

Hammond, S. L., Freimuth, V. S., & Morrison, W. (1987). The gatekeeping funnel: Tracking a major PSA campaign from distribution through gatekeepers to target audience. *Health Education Quarterly, 14,* 153–166.

Harris, D. (1991). AIDS & theory. *Linguafranca, 1*(5), 16–19.

Hyman, H., & Sheatsley, P. (1947). Some reasons why information campaigns fail. *Public Opinion Quarterly, 11,* 412–423.

Kotler, P. (1984). Social marketing of health behavior. In L. W. Frederiksen, L. J. Solomon, & K. A. Brehony (Eds.), *Marketing health behavior* (pp. 23–39). New York: Plenum Press.

Mays, V. M., & Cochran, S. D. (1988). Issues in the perception of AIDS risk and risk reduction activities by black and Hispanic/Latina women. *American Psychologist, 43*(11), 949–957.

McGuire, W. J. (1989). Theoretical foundations of campaigns. In R. E. Rice & C. K. Atkin (Eds.), *Public communication campaigns* (2nd ed., pp. 43–66). Newbury Park, CA: Sage.

McKusick, L., Horstman, W., & Coates, T. (1985). AIDS and sexual behavior reported by gay men in San Francisco. *American Journal of Public Health, 75,* 493–496.

Perloff, R. M., & Pettey, G. (1991). Designing an AIDS information campaign to reach intravenous drug users and sex partners. *Public Health Reports, 106*(4), 460–463.

Petty, R., & Cacioppo, J. (1986). *Communication and persuasion: Central and peripheral routes to attitude change.* New York: Springer-Verlag.

Ray, M. (1973). Marketing communication and the hierarchy of effects. In P. Clark (Ed.), *New models for communication research* (pp. 147–176). Beverly Hills, CA: Sage.

Rogers, E. M. (1983). *Diffusion of innovations* (3rd ed.). New York: The Free Press.

Rogers, E. M., & Storey, J. D. (1987). Communication campaigns. In C. R. Berger & S. H. Chaffee (Eds.), *Handbook of communication science* (pp. 817–846). Newbury Park, CA: Sage.

Salmon, C. T. (1989). Campaigns for social "improvement": An overview of values, rationales, and impacts. In C. T. Salmon (Ed.), *Information campaigns: Balancing social values and social change* (pp. 19–53). Newbury Park, CA: Sage.

Skinner, B. F. (1957). *Verbal behavior.* New York: Appleton-Century-Crofts.

Solomon, D. S. (1989). A social marketing perspective on communication campaigns. In R. E. Rice & C. K. Atkin (Eds.), *Public communication campaigns* (2nd ed., pp. 87–104). Newbury Park, CA: Sage.

U.S. Department of Health and Human Services. (1989). *Making health communication programs work* (NIH Publication No. 89-1493). Bethesda, MD: National Cancer Institute.

Wallack, L. (1990). Mass media and health promotion: Promise, problem, and challenge. In C. Atkin & L. Wallack (Eds.), *Mass communication and public health* (pp. 41–50). Newbury Park, CA: Sage.

Winett, R. A., Altman, D. G., & King, A. C. (1990). Conceptual and strategic foundations for effective media campaigns for preventing the spread of HIV infection. *Evaluation and Program Planning, 13,* 91–104.

CHAPTER SIX

Audience Response to Health Messages About AIDS

Ivana Marková
Kevin Power
University of Stirling, Scotland

The aim of health communicators is to impart knowledge and thus to change health attitudes, perceptions, and health-related behaviors of the audience. However, the impact of health messages on the audience, and the audience's response to such communication, are co-determined by a variety of factors. Among these factors of particular importance are the content of health messages, the personal characteristics and motivation of the audience, and the effect of social environment in which such communication takes place. Although all these factors are important, this chapter focuses on the role of the social environment on health messages. By "social environment" we mean phenomena that in European social science have, for a long time, been explored in terms of "collective representations" (Durkheim, 1898) or "social representations" (Farr & Moscovici, 1984; Jodelet, 1991; Marková & Wilkie, 1987; Moscovici, 1984). Social representations are systems of values, ideas, and practices adopted by members of a particular society; they are the perspectives in terms of which social events are conceptualized and explained. Because people are born into a world of already existing social representations, they adopt them in the same ways that they adopt the other aspects of the physical and social reality.

Social Representations of AIDS

Analyzing the social history of sexually transmitted disease (STD) in the 19th century and first years of the 20th century, Brandt (1985, 1988) drew attention to similarities in the public's fearful responses to AIDS today

111

and those to syphilis and gonorrhea in the early part of this century:

> Theories of casual transmission reflected deep cultural fears about disease
> and sexuality in the early twentieth century. In these approaches to venereal
> disease, concerns about hygiene, contamination, and contagion were ex-
> pressed, anxieties that reflected a great deal about the contemporary soci-
> ety and culture. (Brandt, 1988, p. 367)

Brandt has maintained that STDs were viewed as a threat to the whole
social Victorian system, to its morality and emphasis on self-control. The
ways in which such societal fears and anxieties were expressed at the
time reflect much about the lifestyle, values, and collective images of Victorian society. One can say that the views of Victorian society voiced
a particular *social representation of STDs* prevailing in the existing
culture.

Moscovici (1961/1976, 1984) argued that society forms social representations in order to cope with complex, unfamiliar, and threatening
phenomena. One way of gaining control over such phenomena is to *con-
ventionalize* them. This can be done by *anchoring* them to something
that is already well known and understood. For example, AIDS can be
conventionalized by anchoring it to other STDs.

Thus, social representations are collectively formed and collectively
maintained explanations for events, human activities, and anything else
that cannot easily be fitted within existing schemata. Social representations form the environment within which people think about and conceptualize phenomena and they have a powerful effect on the individual.
Their effect is due to the fact that individuals adopt such representations
unreflectively, being unaware of their effect because they are part of the
sociopsychological environment or social reality in which they live. In
the case of STDs, including AIDS, they encompass not only rational constructs (i.e., the concepts of such diseases), but also societal beliefs and
attitudes, deep-seated socially shared anxieties, cultural values, and moral
norms. The less aware the public is of social representations, the stronger
their effect because they circulate among people unchallenged.

Thus, there is considerable evidence that social representations affect
the ways the public perceives the disease (e.g., Brandt, 1985, 1988; Douglas, 1966; Herzlich & Pierret, 1987). One would expect, therefore, that
such perceptions also affect the way the public responds to health messages. In this chapter we explore whether such questions have been addressed in health communication campaigns and in research. Moreover,
we ask whether health communication campaigns have attempted to
challenge different forms of social representations such as irrational beliefs, values, "old wives tales," and other forms of public knowledge and

social representations. In order to explore these issues we first discuss the main objectives of studies evaluating the efficacy of AIDS programs and point to their limitations. Second, we bring examples, from research, highlighting the interaction between scientific knowledge of HIV/AIDS and social representations. It is argued that the cultural and historical contexts in which AIDS is embedded affect the manner in which an audience actively selects, interprets, and assimilates personally relevant information.

HEALTH COMMUNICATION CAMPAIGNS AND THEIR EVALUATION

Health Communication Campaigns in the United Kingdom

Media-based campaigns are usually funded by central government agencies, and designed to reach large audiences. In contrast, smaller scale health campaigns are often privately funded and are designed for preselected groups. In the United Kingdom the government launched a public AIDS information campaign in 1986. Initially, full-page advertisements in the national press were used to provide facts about HIV and its modes of transmission. Subsequently, cinema, television, radio, and billboard advertisements were used to enhance public awareness about AIDS. In early 1987, a leaflet, entitled "AIDS: Don't Die of Ignorance" was distributed to every household in the country and a national telephone information service was established. This phase is reported to have cost 18 million U.S. dollars. The media-based campaign was deliberately fear provoking, and provided information about the main methods of transmission of HIV and about the groups in society at greatest risk. It implied that the ultimate consequence of AIDS was death. The second phase of the campaign commenced in the Autumn of 1987 with the focus directed on the risks to intravenous drug users (IVDU). In early 1988 another change of emphasis occurred, with the central focus on the risks associated with heterosexual intercourse. It was particularly targeted to young heterosexuals, a group particularly at risk because of the frequency with which they changed sexual partners. Since then, the media campaign has concerned itself with highlighting the risks associated with unprotected homosexual and heterosexual intercourse and with the inherent dangers in sharing unsterilized injecting equipment.

The major objective of this campaign in the United Kingdom has been to improve knowledge of HIV/AIDS, and to increase public awareness of HIV/AIDS because these issues have been assumed to be important precursors for behavior change. Two additional policies have been adopted. First, to encourage those at risk, namely sexually active homosexuals, heterosexuals, and IVDUs, to make the changes in their behavior necessary to prevent the spread of HIV. Second, to convey appropriate information about the ways HIV cannot be transmitted. Such knowledge was considered important to allay any possible public anxiety, to avoid panic concerning HIV/AIDS, and to prevent the stigmatizing of the groups of people at high risk or those who already were HIV antibody positive.

The Effectiveness of Media-Based Campaigns in the United Kingdom

This far-reaching program was very ambitious in wanting to be all things to all people. It is not surprising that there have been contradictory claims regarding the effectiveness of this media-based campaign. Sherr (1987) reported that the governmental health communication slightly increased public knowledge but had no effect on adjusting misconceptions about HIV/AIDS and did not lower public anxiety. In addition, attitudes of fear, outrage, and sympathy remained unaltered, and sexual behavior itself was unchanged. In general, Sherr found the results of the campaign disappointing. In a similar way, Nutbeam, Catford, Smail, and Griffiths (1989) reported that although the campaign seemed effective in improving knowledge about the key methods of transmission and about the groups at greatest risk, considerable misunderstandings about HIV/AIDS have still persisted among a large proportion of the general public. In addition, the level of ignorance was closely related to attitudes indicative of prejudice. The authors concluded that

> it is disappointing that understanding has remained so limited in many people following such a major public information campaign. The anxieties that have remained may well have unwarranted effects on individuals . . . and may also lead to unjustified discrimination against people with AIDS. (p. 210)

The authors maintained that "measures to combat AIDS in Britain have, so far, informed but not educated the public" (p. 210). A rather different conclusion was reported by Wober (1988) who found that general self-assessed or personally claimed knowledge rose considerably over the 10-week period of the campaign and that there was a positive correlation between claimed and tested knowledge. In other words, those who acquired more AIDS-related knowledge also regarded themselves as more knowledgeable, most of all at the time of the post-campaign assessment, which was immediately after a 10-week period of health communication campaign. Wober concluded that although the campaign contributed to the increase in knowledge, it was not obvious whether this had any behavioral or attitudinal consequences. Finally, Mills, Campbell, and Waters (1986) evaluated the media campaign between February and June 1986. Contrary to other researchers, they found that there was a decrease in public knowledge of AIDS over this period. A further study by Campbell and Waters (1987) compared their June 1986 results with those obtained in December 1986 after another extensive media campaign. In contrast to the previous study, the results from the latter research indicated a small increase in overall AIDS-related knowledge. It was found that more people than before realized that the infection could not be caught by sharing eating and drinking utensils with those infected by HIV. However, there was still considerable public uncertainty as to whether AIDS could be transmitted by blood or blood products and whether donated blood was tested for the presence of HIV. The authors concluded that further public health communication concerning AIDS was necessary.

Difficulties in Assessing the Campaign

The question arises as to why there should be such discrepant conclusions as to the success or failure of these vast and expensive media campaigns in the United Kingdom. There are a number of factors that might affect the outcome of their evaluation. First, the time of the collection of the data obviously influences results. One can expect that the longer the time period between pre- and posttesting and the greater the amount of information presented between these times, the greater the likelihood of significant increases in knowledge. Second, the comparison of knowledge between 1985 when the general level of public information was presumably low and 1988, after the main government campaigns, could have led to more statistically significant results with respect to increased knowledge than the comparison between 1988 and 1991. In the latter case, a ceiling or saturation effect may have diminished the likelihood of finding a significant increase in knowledge over time. Third, the size and characteristics of the population sample would be expected to influence results. For example, Sherr's (1987) sample consisted of 159 high-risk and 83 low-risk participants at pretest and 107 high-risk and 76 low-risk participants at posttest. In contrast, Wober's (1988) study involved 1,001 and 1,004 participants at pre- and posttest, respectively. Unfortunately, studies investigating the efficacy of media-based campaigns can seldom select the same subject panel at pre- and posttest assessments, which may therefore compromise the validity of the results. Fourth, the type and amount of the assessed educational material differs from one study to another, thereby preventing interstudy comparisons. Fifth, in such studies it is difficult to control for extraneous educational input and for the participants' experience. Moreover, it is difficult to obtain a control group that is not subjected to mass media and other educational programs. Sixth, and probably most important, different studies appear to use different criteria for determining success or failure of the media-based health campaigns. Some reports (Wellings & McVey, 1990; White et al., 1988) have suggested that raising awareness of HIV/AIDS is an essential criterion for determining success. Other studies (Campbell & Waters, 1987; Wober, 1988) assume that knowledge of HIV/AIDS is a suitable yardstick for measuring the effectiveness of campaigns. Results of such studies obviously differ, depending on the number of items included in their knowledge examination and on the degree of specificity or difficulty attached to such knowledge items. Other studies use changes in sexual behavior as a determinant of outcome (Emmons et al., 1986) and still others focus on attitude change or anxiety reduction (Nutbeam et al., 1989). As it is likely that it is more difficult to change sexual behavior than to increase awareness of HIV/AIDS, the dependent outcome measure chosen by health communication evaluators will surely influence their final conclusions about the effectiveness of a campaign.

Another problem in assessing the impact of national health campaigns is that the public does not comprise a homogeneous group. Different groups, such as homosexuals, heterosexuals, IVDUs, monogamous and polygamous individuals, adolescents, adults, the elderly, and the recipients of blood products, are subject to different risks and are likely to have different educational needs. Government media campaigns, trying to address "everybody" at the same time, are unlikely to be able to respond to this diversity of need. In addition, some aspects of the early media campaign seem rather contradictory. For example, the attempts to change behavior by inducing fear seem at odds with the attempts to reduce irrational anxieties and fears of contagion by social contact. The presentation of AIDS as a feature of certain groups, such as homosexuals and IVDUs, is likely to induce discrimination and stigmatization. Moreover, it may magnify negative, irrational attitudes rather than foster social acceptance and support for those who are HIV antibody positive.

Health Communication
for Preselected At-Risk Groups

A number of researchers worldwide have attempted to evaluate health messages that are planned, implemented, and targeted to meet the specific needs of certain individuals. For example, investigations have included those who might have excessive anxiety and concerns regarding their personal susceptibility to the virus or those who were at risk by virtue of their behavioral patterns. We briefly refer to the studies that have been carried out in different parts of the world and to evaluative programs targeted at specific groups.

Despite the very small risk of HIV transmission to health workers, they have been subject to misconceptions, ignorance, and prejudice regarding contact with HIV antibody positive patients. Research on the evaluation of communication programs for health workers has shown that with increased knowledge of HIV/AIDS the perceived risk to the self decreases and more positive attitudes toward infected patients are formed (Armstrong-Esther & Hewitt, 1990; Brattebø, Wisborg, & Sjursen, 1990; McKinnon, Insall, Gooch, & Cockcroft, 1990; O'Donnell & O'Donnell, 1987).

Studies of health communication programs for young heterosexuals in elementary schools, high schools, and colleges have been undertaken with a range of aims. Some studies have asked such basic questions as whether the educational programs offered were "helpful" (Scott, Chambers, Underwood, Walter, & Pickard, 1990). Other studies have concentrated on assessing changes in knowledge and attitudes after participation in educational programs (Brown, Fritz, & Barone, 1989; Chandarana, Conlon, Noh, & Field, 1990; Clift & Stears, 1988; DiClemente et al., 1989; Gillian & Seltzer, 1989; Rhodes & Wolitski, 1989). Yet other studies have explored knowledge and specific attitudes regarding willingness to practice risk-reducing behaviors (Huszti, Clopton, & Mason, 1989). Finally, Hernandez and Smith (1990) assessed the impact of education intervention on older adolescents' attitudes and behavior regarding sex and dating. It appears that educational approaches among young heterosexuals improve awareness and increase knowledge of HIV/AIDS. Some authors found no change regarding AIDS-related attitudes (Rhodes & Wolitski, 1989), whereas others reported greater tolerance of AIDS patients and more hesitation about high-risk behaviors (Brown et al., 1989; Di Clemente et al., 1989). However, hesitation about high-risk behavior does not necessarily mean willingness to adopt satisfactory risk-reducing behavior. Huszti et al. (1989) found that although health messages increase knowledge and positive attitudes toward patients with AIDS, they do not appear to have a positive effect on attitudes toward practicing sexual behaviors that would prevent the spread of HIV. The authors concluded that more intensive programs may be necessary to effect behavioral change.

Hernandez and Smith (1990) have investigated the impact of three communication approaches on cognitive factors (e.g., on sexual motivation in dating and intention to use condoms), and on sex-related behaviors (e.g., frequency of condom use and number of sex partners). The three approaches, each comprising educational literature and a video, were selected to represent the types of programs advocated by boards of education, health organizations, and health educators. They included the following: (a) a program presenting sex abstinence as the best and only certain prevention strategy; (b) a "decision-making" program presenting safer sex and describing it as an alternative to abstinence; and (c) a "protection" program presenting abstinence as the safest alternative and safe sex the second best. In addition, the third program explicitly described how to use condoms and how to negotiate safer sex with partners. The behavioral response to the health communication programs was complex. Although all three reported a greater intention to use condoms, an increase in carrying condoms and a decrease in the likelihood of sex abstinence, there were no differences between them in condom use, sex abstinence, monogamy, or delay of sex for precautionary reasons. However, there were differences between males/females and sexually active/inactive people on a number of cognitive and behavioral factors. The differences illustrate that the impact of education programs will vary with individual differences in the composition of the audience.

A small number of studies have attempted to elucidate the factors that may lead to risk-reducing behaviors among homosexual and bisexual males. Although no differences between several communication approaches were found when "safer sex" was measured globally, it was found that these approaches had a differential effect on certain subcategories of "safer sex," such as condom usage, monogamy, and avoidance of anal intercourse (Robert & Rosser, 1990). On the basis of this study, the authors argued that any evaluations of AIDS education programs must take into consideration the diversity of safer-sex practices and the differential impact of communication approaches on them. Valdiserri and his co-workers (1987) emphasized the importance of peer norms and of social context in health-related behavior and they argued that these must be part of any health education program. In their subsequent work, Valdiserri et al. (1989) found that the inclusion of a skills training component covering the promotion of social acceptability and the legitimacy of safer sex led to changes in specific self-reported sexual behaviors. The authors argued that techniques that teach homosexual men to negotiate and to rehearse safer sexual encounters can result in benefits over and above the mere dissemination of information. Their emphasis on "self-empowerment" illustrates the personal efficacy of adopting, developing, and implementing a rational risk reduction technique that is related to personal risk but is approved and sanctioned by prior peer-group acceptability. It is necessary to add, however, that even when behavioral changes are implemented, they do not necessarily apply to all sexual activities but may only influence specific practices.

There is a dearth of studies concerning the efficacy of educational programs to alter injecting practices among IVDUs. Jackson, Rotkiewicz,

Quinones, and Passannante (1989) reported a 1-hour AIDS communication program, provided on a one-to-one basis either by an ex-addict or by a professional AIDS counsellor, dealing with transmission, safer sex, and IVDU risk reduction. Although little hard data was presented, the authors concluded that IVDUs' knowledge of AIDS increased after participation in the program.

Recently, attention has focused on health education in prisons, due to suspected homosexuality and drug use. Conolly (1989) reported that inmates who had received AIDS educational lectures or literature were more knowledgeable about HIV/AIDS than those who had received no information. However, there was no difference between "educated" and "noneducated" prisoners' attitudes about AIDS. Over 70% of prisoners believed that segregation and compulsory AIDS testing to identify HIV antibody positive prisoners would help to stop the spread of AIDS. Exploring knowledge of HIV/AIDS, attitudes toward those infected with HIV and the perception of risk of HIV in Scottish prisons, Power, Marková, and Rowlands (1991) have examined the efficacy of the educational video made by the Department of Health and Social Security in the United Kingdom. This video was particularly prepared for prisoners, as was a similar version for prison officers. It first shows the immunodeficiency virus as an object moving in spatiotemporal configurations with respect to the white blood cells. It then shows it penetrating white cells, demolishing them, and eventually suppressing and destroying the body's defenses. It depicts a number of scenes, such as a young woman and a young man meeting in a pub and, after drinking from the same glass, going to a flat and having sexual intercourse, and the question as to whether they should use a condom is raised. There are scenes in the video involving intercourse between two homosexual men, then between lesbians; there is also a violent scene in a prison, scenes with drug users, and finally a person infected with HIV and her desperate future. The purpose of the film is to educate viewers as to how HIV is transmitted, and what is and is not a risk behavior. It was found that the main difference between the group of 323 prisoners who saw the video and 236 who did not see it was that those who saw it were more knowledgeable about the lack of risk associated with social/casual contact. However, there was a tendency for the prisoners who saw the video to be more homophobic in their attitudes.

Problems of the Evaluative Studies

In previous sections we have tried to show that from the beginning of the AIDS epidemic, the emphasis has been put on increase in knowledge, alteration of attitudes, reduction of anxiety, and change of risk-taking behavior of individuals. Much less attention has been paid to the socio-historical and cultural contexts of health education that might generate such attitudes, beliefs, and representations of HIV/AIDS and to the personal relevance of health-related messages.

Most of these evaluative studies are based on a particular kind of individualistic philosophy that conceptualizes human beings as rational information-processing systems. These studies largely ignore the fact that people assimilate provided information actively and selectively on the basis of relevant personal and societal factors, and that these factors interplay with each other. For example, past experience, mood, perceived risk, social norms, representations, and beliefs, are all decisive in people's assimilation of available information. The intelligibility and manner in which health communication is delivered may therefore affect the understanding and memory of, and compliance with, the message.

A further problem with research concerning *knowledge, attitudes, awareness,* and *sexual behavior* is lack of conceptual clarity of these terms. Knowledge of AIDS may apply to a host of separate issues, such as modes of transmission, epidemiological issues, methods of prevention, risk behaviors, and so on. Attitudes may refer, for example, to willingness to adopt safer sex, propensity to stigmatize those with HIV/AIDS, support for coercive screening measures, and to homophobia. Awareness is applied to memory of having seen AIDS advertisements, to acceptability of the needs of HIV antibody positive individuals, and to the level of AIDS-related knowledge. Moreover, it is evident that terms such as *knowledge, attitudes,* and *awareness* have at times been used synonymously and in an overlapping fashion. Moreover, *sexual behavior* and *safer sex* refer to a range of activities that may be differentially affected by educational interventions.

SOCIAL REPRESENTATIONS AND KNOWLEDGE OF HIV/AIDS

In addition to problems due to terminological ambiguity, there is also a problem arising from different modes of knowing something about AIDS. At the one end of the spectrum there is knowing in a strictly scientific sense. Such knowing is characterized by impartiality, and social values are not part of it. It is concerned with explicit facts that are publicly available in scientific journals or in information leaflets.

At the other end of the spectrum is the social representational knowing that we introduced earlier in this chapter. It is the kind of knowing that is collectively constructed by a particular society and it circulates among people through "old wives tales," beliefs, rumors, and through semiconscious and unconscious associations. Much of this knowing is implicit, which means that people are often not aware of its existence. Some of this knowing is supported by evidence. This kind of knowing lives through the culture and is often transmitted from generation to generation. The beginning of the AIDS epidemic in the early 1980s was characterized by a phase with virtually no scientific knowledge of AIDS. Yet the public responded to AIDS instantly by applying social representations that have existed in Western culture for centuries and have been associated with sex pollution, immorality, the punishment of sinners, and with public danger due to outcasts (Brandt, 1985, 1988; Douglas, 1966).

The Personal Relevance of Health Education Messages

The knowledge that one is or may be at risk of infection by HIV is not neutral with respect to oneself but is personally relevant. In other words, it is unlikely that the individual assimilates such knowledge in a purely objective manner. Rather, such knowledge is a threatening piece of self-information that induces emotional response. Therefore, advertisements, information in leaflets, and posters may be interpreted in different ways by different individuals and at-risk groups.

Stockdale and Farr (1987) and Stockdale, Dockrell, and Wells (1989) have studied the messages conveyed by AIDS posters targeted either at homosexuals or heterosexuals. The respondents were asked to answer a number of open-ended questions about the posters, for example, what they thought the main message was and at whom they thought the poster was aimed. They also rated the posters on personal relevance, relevance to the majority of the population, clarity, impact, creation of fear, provision of new information, the interest they generated, and whether people were likely to change their behavior as a result of viewing the poster. The authors found considerable differences between perceptions of posters by homosexuals and by heterosexuals. The posters targeted at the homosexual community were perceived in a more positive manner by homosexuals than by heterosexuals. For example, although homosexuals tended to describe a particular poster as "warm and loving," "sensual," and commending one to "take care of the one you love," the heterosexuals described it as "stark and sad." Overall, the study showed that the representations of HIV/AIDS held by homosexuals and heterosexuals are fundamental to their perceptions of educational materials. The authors argued that it is pointless to present educational materials that aim a message at everyone because this does not provide an adequate reference group for the individual to examine his or her own behavior. The efficacy of campaigns may well depend on the proper targeting of the at-risk groups.

Kitzinger (in press) has explored the perceptions of the poster "two eyes–nose–mouth" (see Fig. 6.1) used in the United Kingdom as a health warning about HIV/AIDS. This poster was intended to convey the message that it is impossible to identify a person with HIV by his or her appearance and therefore one should always take precautions when having sex. Although the majority of participants claimed that HIV infection is not visible to the naked eye, when referring to their day-to-day experiences some participants said that they indeed used a person's appearance to decide whether or not he or she was HIV antibody positive. Different groups of people, including doctors, social workers, prisoners, male prostitutes, heterosexual men, and gay men were all able to describe "safe-looking" versus "unsafe-looking" patients, clients, or lovers (Kitzinger, in press). Some adolescents and rent boys (young male prostitutes) thought that by looking into a person's eyes, or at his or her nose and mouth, one can actually discover whether the person is infected by HIV, for example: "Aye, their eyes are all black underneath," "the eyes are all dazzly," "frothy at the mouth," or "look at their eyes, look at their nose and look at their mouth and if they look queer you dunnae bother going near them," reasons very different from those intended by the designer. The interviewees maintained that by looking into a person's eyes, at his or her nose and mouth, you can actually discover whether the person is infected by HIV because this is, they thought, where it shows (Kitzinger & Beharrell, 1990).

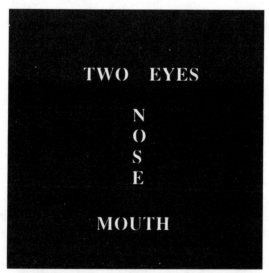

HOW TO RECOGNIZE SOMEONE WITH HIV.

FIG. 6.1. The "two eyes–nose–mouth" poster used in the United Kingdom as a health warning about HIV/AIDS.

Rhodes and Wolitski (1989) assessed viewers' ratings of AIDS educational videos on several dimensions:

1. effectiveness in communicating information,
2. effectiveness in addressing personal concerns about AIDS,
3. ability to hold viewers' attention,
4. realism,
5. clarity, and
6. possible offensiveness of the presentation.

It was found that those videos rated by viewers as most appealing also produced greatest gains in knowledge and changes in attitudes. Moreover, the data suggested that personal concerns of viewers, clarity, and ability to hold attention increase the effectiveness of videos. Hastings, Leather, and Scott (1987) used qualitative small-group discussions of heterosexuals, homosexuals, and drug addicts to evaluate an AIDS leaflet designed for "everyone." A sample of 84 individuals recruited from the general public all perceived the leaflet as targeted at at-risk groups only. Neither homosexuals nor drug addicts saw the leaflet as personally relevant or having direct implications for their own sexual behavior. On the basis of these findings, the leaflet was changed before it was distributed. The authors concluded that without this form of consumer research appropriate changes could not have been made to the leaflet and that the leaflet would not only have been ineffective but also counterproductive.

Knowledge of HIV/AIDS and the Fear of Stigma

Between 1981 and 1985 a considerable proportion of people with a severe form of hemophilia, a genetic disorder of blood clotting, who treated their bleedings with a commercially produced factor obtained from blood, were infected with HIV. They therefore did not conceive of HIV as a sexually transmitted infection but as an infection spread through blood. Indeed, some patients found it difficult to understand the transmission of infection. For example, in research carried out in Scotland in 1986–1987, one person with hemophilia commented that he "understood that HIV could be spread by semen because he had been told" but he found this difficult to believe because "people with hemophilia get HIV from the blood, and so how does the blood get into the semen?" (Marková, Wilkie, & Forbes, 1988). At the time of this research it was believed in the United Kingdom that there should be no differential treatment of patients with hemophilia who were HIV antibody positive and those who were antibody negative. The reason for this was to maintain the confidentiality of those who were HIV antibody positive. The advice to patients in most hemophilia centers was to practice safer sex and to have no children. This nondifferential treatment led to a problem for those who were HIV antibody negative because they received, simultaneously, two different kinds of message. On the one hand they were to believe that the blood products needed for treatment of their bleedings were entirely safe because blood donors were screened for the presence of HIV and blood products were heat treated to destroy any remaining HIV. A patient with hemophilia who was HIV antibody negative and had not received contaminated blood was therefore no more at risk of HIV than any other heterosexual person. Therefore, the advice these patients received, that they should not have children, was difficult to square with the information that they were entirely free of infection. From the point of view of the medical staff, however, it was equally difficult to provide individualized information without breaching the confidentiality of the patient. Thus, under such conditions, medical staff encountered problems to which there could be no "right" or "wrong" solutions. This example highlights the point that the same educational message given to different at-risk groups may be understandable in one case but confusing in another.

Of the 40 sexually active male patients with hemophilia who participated in the Scottish research (Marková, Wilkie, Naji, & Forbes, 1990a), only 15 (38%) reported using condoms. The failure to use condoms, however, was not due to the patients not knowing the risk to their partners (Marková, Wilkie, Naji, & Forbes, 1990b). Rather, their comments in interviews with the counsellor indicated that they found it extremely difficult to cope with their situation because of the stigma attached to HIV/AIDS and therefore of the fear that they, themselves, might become stigmatized. We explain this problem by considering such difficulties for different groups of patients with hemophilia. For patients in stable relationships, the use of condoms was often associated with dirt. AIDS was considered a sexually transmitted "dirty disease." In addition, several patients with hemophilia said that they did not tell their wives that they were at risk of HIV infection. These wives understood and did not ask questions. The use of a condom would have meant spelling out the issue of concern and the couples did not have the courage to do this. Those who had never had a sexual partner, such as 16- to 20-year-olds, assumed that most girls were on the pill, and therefore would question the use of a condom. One young man, without a regular girlfriend, who had learned that he was HIV antibody positive, pointed out that many girls used their own contraception and were unlikely to see the need for additional protection. Indeed, when he had on one occasion produced a condom he had been asked whether there was something wrong with him or whether he had AIDS. Another patient said that to tell his girlfriend that he was HIV antibody positive was just too difficult. He questioned whether a girl would wish to remain in a relationship with someone who had HIV. Only one young patient developed a positive strategy. He used a condom and explained this to his partner in the following way: "I am into the rubber. It turns me on." However, such an attitude was an exception. Some patients with hemophilia in a similar situation tended not to form any long-term relationships that would commit them to explaining their HIV antibody status to their partners. They tended to drift from one relationship to another and satisfied themselves with one-night stands, which, they thought, did not require any explanation to the girl. It appears from a number of patients' comments that their main reason for not using a condom was their anxiety of being rejected by others if they revealed their HIV antibody positive status.

Several respondents said that their HIV antibody status was a confidential matter and they did not wish others to know about it. Some of those who were HIV antibody negative said they did not mind who knew, but that it would be very different should they become HIV antibody positive. Of 59 patients, 45 (76%) implied or explicitly stated that they were concerned about the stigmatizing effect of HIV infection and AIDS. Thirteen patients (20%) said that they would not reveal their HIV antibody status even to their sexual partners (Marková et al., 1990b).

Knowledge of HIV/AIDS and the Fear of Contagion

Although at the time of the study (Marková et al., 1990b), most patients and their parents either knew or were told at the time that household contacts did not present a risk of HIV/AIDS, they associated HIV and AIDS with uncleanliness. For example, one mother said that she had "spent a small fortune on bleach since she knew about HIV." She was very concerned that nobody should think that she kept a "dirty house." Another mother admitted that she poured disinfectant down the toilet after her son had been there. Indeed, the word "dirty" was raised on many occasions. An association of HIV infection with dirt can also be inferred from the following example. One hundred and four members of medical, paramedical, and clerical hospital staff, who had participated in the Scottish hemophilia study, were also interviewed on their knowledge of HIV/AIDS. Although most of the interviewees gave correct answers about the transmission of HIV infection, 42 (40%) of them, including 3 doctors, thought that persons with HIV should be barred from working in the food industry and from professions in which food handling is required (Marková et al., 1988).

The associations, by patients, their families, and medical and paramedical staff, of HIV/AIDS with dirt is reminiscent of the study of Jodelet

(1991). Her study was based on observations of villagers in France who offered their homes to ex-patients from mental hospitals. Although voluntarily responding to the governmental call and inviting these ex-patients as paying guests into their homes, the villagers devised ingenious strategies to isolate themselves from them. For example, they rescheduled their mealtimes so that they would not eat with them, washed their laundry separately, used different kinds of crockery, and did not allow their daughters to become too friendly with these ex-patients with a history of mental illness. Thus, although the villagers made a rational decision to accept these ex-patients, their implicitly shared fear of contagion of mental illness through personal closeness led them to adopt irrational activities. In a similar vein, Sontag (1989) referred to perceived contagion of illnesses and to irrational and implicit beliefs with respect to AIDS.

TOWARD MORE COMPREHENSIVE HEALTH MESSAGES

The public response to AIDS has shown the unfading strength of unconsciously shared collective representations of the disease, such as fears, anxieties, beliefs, and myths that have survived in our society for many centuries. It appears that Douglas' (1966) approach to the study of culture is pertinent here. According to Douglas, natural objects and artifacts are viewed by people on the dimension clean–dirty and classified accordingly. Events and actions that pollute things are associated with disorder and immorality. What is clean and dirty, sacred and holy, or pure and polluted, where and when, is a matter of symbolic systems in given cultures. Taking this approach to culture, disease and illness has traditionally been associated with social scourge, punishment of sins, impurity, stigma, and consequently with the exclusion of the sick and ill from society for fear of contagion (Herzlich & Pierret, 1984/1987). The fears and worries of patients with hemophilia and their families with respect to HIV/AIDS that were discussed earlier in this chapter express the representations and associations to which Douglas (1966) and Herzlich and Pierret (1984/1987) referred.

The fact that health communication has remained unaffected by the insights of sociology, social anthropology, and the social history of science into the collective and social representations of the disease, and that it has been almost exclusively information- and knowledge-based, is itself a fascinating cultural phenomenon. We have shown that the philosophy underlying the majority of health communication campaigns concerning HIV/AIDS has been information- and knowledge-based. In contrast, research has indicated that social and collective representations of

HIV/AIDS may have a stronger effect on people's behavior than the scientifically based knowledge. The personal relevance of health communication and sociocultural factors may strongly affect an audience's response to health communication. It should be acknowledged by those responsible for health campaigns that information and knowledge are never constructed by consumers as neutral. Rather, information about the disease and knowledge of the disease are always conceived in the context of some relationship to the self and society. It is clear that to increase the efficacy of HIV/AIDS educational messages, it is essential to close the gap between the philosophy on which the present health communication campaigns are based and the assumptions of the underlying theory of social representations. We suggest that this could be achieved by a more comprehensive approach to health communication.

Health communication needs to address the discrepancy between adequate levels of HIV/AIDS knowledge and inadequate levels of behavioral risk reduction. Valdiserri et al. (1987) have shown that changes of attitudes toward high-risk sexual behavior are best achieved in small-group discussions. This method permits modification of peer-group norms of what is socially acceptable sexual behavior, provides social support for behavioral risk reduction, alters irrational beliefs and attitudes, and personalizes the need for behavioral change. Homans and Aggleton (1988) have supported the opinion that such methods are also more effective than impersonal mass media campaigns, because they impart information by word of mouth and personal contact.

Perception of risk also depends on the individual's own self-perception and self-categorization. For example, in Stockdale et al.'s (1989) study, homosexuals perceived themselves as being in stable relationships and thus less at risk than those heterosexuals who were not in stable relationships. Heterosexuals, however, stereotyped homosexuals, bisexuals, and IVDUs as being most at risk from HIV. Stockdale (1990) pointed out that despite the fact that only about half of her heterosexual respondents were in stable relationships, they identified with heterosexuals in such relationships, distancing themselves from those whom they perceived to be at risk. It thus appears that the individual's response to health education campaigns also depends on his or her view of him or herself in relation to at-risk groups.

The results of the studies evaluating the effectiveness of health communication messages in HIV/AIDS have drawn attention to the complexities of the communication process. In particular, one can infer that scientific and public knowledge of HIV/AIDS cannot easily be integrated because these two kinds of knowledge have different aims (Marková, 1991). Thus, campaigns presenting factual scientific knowledge of HIV/AIDS call for rational and responsible behavior so that the disease does not spread. Public or social representational knowledge, on the other hand, focuses the individual's attention on stigma and rejection by others, and therefore calls for actions that do not reveal an individual's HIV antibody status.

Because AIDS is still perceived by the public as a fundamentally stigmatizing disease, health communication concerning HIV/AIDS will have to address and respond to not only the audience's perceptions, knowledge, and attitudes but also the underlying sociocultural assumptions and social representations on which such perceptions, knowledge, and attitudes are based.

REFERENCES

Armstrong-Esther, C., & Hewitt, W. E. (1990). The effect of education on nurses' perception of AIDS. *Journal of Advanced Nursing, 15,* 638–651.

Brandt, A. M. (1985). *No magic bullet.* Oxford: Oxford University Press.

Brandt, A. M. (1988). AIDS in historical perspective: Four lessons from the history of sexually transmitted diseases. *American Journal of Public Health, 78,* 367–371.

Brattebø, G., Wisborg, T., & Sjursen, H. (1990). Health workers and the human immunodeficiency virus: Knowledge, ignorance and behaviour. *Public Health, 104,* 123–130.

Brown, L. K., Fritz, G. K., & Barone, V. J. (1989). The impact of AIDS education on junior and senior high school students. *Journal of Adolescent Health Care, 10,* 386–392.

Campbell, M. J., & Waters, W. E. (1987). Public knowledge about AIDS increasing. *British Medical Journal, 294,* 892–893.

Chandarana, P. C., Conlon, P., Noh, S., & Field, V. A. (1990). The impact of AIDS education among elementary school students. *Canadian Journal of Public Health, 81,* 286–289.

Clift, S. M., & Stears, D. F. (1988). Beliefs and attitudes regarding AIDS among British college students: A preliminary study of change between November 1986 and May 1987. *Health Education Research, 3,* 75–88.

Conolly, L. (1989). Evaluation of the AIDS education program for prisoners in the N.S.W. Department of Corrective Services: March 1987 to March 1989. *Department of Corrective Services Research Publication, 20.*

DiClemente, R. J., Pies, C. A., Stoller, E. M., Straits, C., Olivia, G. E., Haskin, J., & Rutherford, G. W. (1989). Evaluation of school-based AIDS education curricula in San Francisco. *The Journal of Sex Research, 26,* 188–198.

Douglas, M. (1966). *Purity and danger.* London: Routledge & Kegan Paul.

Durkheim, E. (1898). Représentations individuelles et représentations collectives [Individual representations and collective representations]. *Revue de Métaphysique et de Morale, VI,* 273–302.

Emmons, C-A., Joseph, J. G., Kessler, R. C., Wortman, C. B., Montgomery, S. B., & Ostrow, D. G. (1986). Psychosocial predictors of reported behavior change in homosexual men and risk for AIDS. *Health Education Quarterly, 13,* 331–345.

Farr, R. M., & Moscovici, S. (Eds.). (1984). *Social representations.* Cambridge: Cambridge University Press.

Gillian, A., & Seltzer, R. (1989). The efficacy of educational movies on AIDS knowledge and attitudes among college students. *College Health, 37,* 261–265.

Hastings, G. B., Leather, D. S., & Scott, A. C. (1987). AIDS publicity: Some experiences from Scotland. *British Medical Journal, 294,* 48–49.

Hernandez, J. T., & Smith, F. J. (1990). Abstinence, protection, and decision-making: Experimental trials on prototypic AIDS programs. *Health Education Research, 5,* 309–320.

Herzlich, C., & Pierret, J. (1987). *Illness and self in society* (E. Forster, Trans.). Baltimore, MD: The Johns Hopkins University Press. (Original work published 1984)

Homans, H., & Aggleton, P. (1988). Health education, HIV infection and AIDS. In P. Aggleton & H. Homans (Eds.), *Social aspects of AIDS* (pp. 154–176). London: Falmer Press.

Huszti, H. C., Clopton, J. R., & Mason, P. J. (1989). Acquired immunodeficiency syndrome educational program: Effects on adolescents' knowledge and attitudes. *Pediatrics, 84,* 986–994.

Jackson, J. F., Rotkiewicz, L. G., Quinones, M. A., & Passannante, M. R. (1989). A coupon program—drug treatment and AIDS education. *The International Journal of the Addictions, 24,* 1035–1051.

Jodelet, D. (1991). *Madness and social representations.* Hemel Hempstead: Harvester Wheatsheaf.

Kitzinger, J. (in press). Judging by appearances: Audience understandings of "the look" of someone with HIV. *Journal of Community and Applied Social Psychology.*

Kitzinger, J., & Beharrell, P. (1990, March). *Audience responses to media messages on AIDS/ HIV.* Paper presented at the conference on Attitudes, Behaviours and HIV Infection, Royal College of Physicians, The Scottish Home and Health Department, Edinburgh, Scotland.

Marková, I. (1991). Scientific and public knowledge of AIDS: The problem of their integration. In M. von Cranach, W. Doise, & G. Mugny (Eds.), *Social representations and the social bases of knowledge* (pp. 179–183). Bern: Huber.

Marková, I., & Wilkie, P. A. (1987). Representations, concepts and social change: The phenomenon of AIDS. *Journal for the Theory of Social Behaviour, 17,* 389–407.

Marková, I., Wilkie, P. A., & Forbes, C. D. (1988). *Coping strategies of hemophilic patients who are at risk from acquired immunity deficiency syndrome (AIDS) and implications for counselling.* Unpublished final report to the Scottish Home and Health Department.

Marková, I., Wilkie, P. A., Naji, S. A., & Forbes, C. D. (1990a). Self- and other-awareness of the risk of HIV/AIDS in people with hemophilia and implications for behavioural change. *Social Science and Medicine, 31,* 73–79.

Marková, I., Wilkie, P. A., Naji, S. A., & Forbes, C. D. (1990b). Knowledge of HIV/AIDS and behavioural change of people with hemophilia. *Psychology and Health, 4,* 125–133.

McKinnon, M. D., Insall, C., Gooch, C. D., & Cockcroft, A. (1990). Knowledge and attitudes of health care workers about AIDS and infection before and after distribution of an educational booklet. *Journal of Social Occupation Medicine, 40,* 15–18.

Mills, S., Campbell, M. J., & Waters, W. E. (1986). Public knowledge of AIDS and the DHSS advertisement campaign. *British Medical Journal, 293,* 1089–1090.

Moscovici, S. (1976). *La psychanalyse: Son image et son public* [Psychoanalysis: Its image and public distribution]. Paris: Presses Universitaire de France. (Original work published 1961)

Moscovici, S. (1984). The phenomenon of social representations. In R. M. Farr & S. Moscovici (Eds.), *Social representations* (pp. 3–69). Cambridge: Cambridge University Press.

Nutbeam, D., Catford, J. C., Smail, S. A., & Griffiths, C. (1989). Public knowledge and attitudes to AIDS. *Public Health, 103,* 205–211.

O'Donnell, L., & O'Donnell, C. R. (1987). Hospital workers and AIDS: Effect of in-service education on knowledge and perceived risks and stresses. *New York State Journal of Medicine, 87,* 279–289.

Power, K. G., Marková, I., & Rowlands, A. (1991). *HIV/AIDS knowledge, attitudes, and personal risk in the Scottish prison service.* Unpublished final report to the Scottish Home and Health Department, Edinburgh.

Rhodes, F., & Wolitski, R. (1989). Effect of instructional videotapes on AIDS knowledge and attitudes. *College Health, 37,* 266–271.

Robert, B., & Rosser, S. (1990). Evaluation of the efficacy of AIDS education interventions for homosexually active men. *Health Education Research, 5,* 299–308.

Scott, F., Chambers, L. W., Underwood, J., Walter, S., & Pickard, L. (1990). AIDS seminars for senior grades in secondary schools. *Canadian Journal of Public Health, 81,* 290–294.

Sherr, L. (1987). An evaluation of UK government health education campaign on AIDS. *Psychology and Health, 1,* 61–72.

Sontag, S. (1989). *AIDS and its metaphors.* London: The Penguin Press.

Stockdale, J. E., Dockrell, J. E., & Wells, A. J. (1989). The self in relation to mass media representations of HIV and AIDS: Match or mismatch? *Health Education Journal, 48,* 121–130.

Stockdale, J. E., & Farr, R. M. (1987, December). *Social representation of handicap in poster campaigns.* Paper presented at the London Conference of The British Psychological Society, London.

Stockdale, J. E. (1990, August). *The self and media messages: Match or mismatch?* Paper presented at the British Association of the Advancement of Science, Swansea.

Valdiserri, R. O., Lyter, D. W., Kingsley, L. A., Leviton, L. C., Schofield, J. W., Huggins, J., Ho, M., & Rinaldo, C. R. (1987). The effect of group education on improving attitudes about AIDS risk reduction. *New York State Journal of Medicine, 87,* 272–278.

Valdiserri, R. O., Lyter, D. W., Leviton, L. C., Callahan, C. M., Kingsley, L. A., & Rinaldo, C. R. (1989). AIDS prevention in homosexual and bisexual men: Results of a randomized trial evaluating two risk reduction interventions. *Current Science, 3,* 21–26.

Wellings, K., & McVey, D. (1990). Evaluation of the HEA AIDS press campaign: December 1988 to March 1989. *Health Education Journal, 49,* 108–116.

White, D. G., Phillips, K. C., Pitts, M., Clifford, B. R., Elliott, J. R., & Davies, M. M. (1988). Adolescents' perceptions of AIDS. *Health Education Journal, 47,* 117–119.

Wober, J. M. (1988). Informing the British public about AIDS. *Health Education Research, 3,* 19–24.

CHAPTER SEVEN

A Systems Approach to AIDS Communication: The Example of the National AIDS Information and Education Program

Charles T. Salmon
University of Wisconsin

Fred Kroger
Centers for Disease Control

The individual has been the unit of analysis for a considerable number of studies and treatises on communication effects and concomitant processes of social change. This orientation has been important, as all change efforts necessarily involve individuals at some point, especially as discrete "targets" of educational and persuasive messages. In the specific arena of health communication, researchers have developed or adapted (from cognitive and social psychology) several theoretical models of individual-level change. These models, in turn, have been applied in numerous communication campaigns designed to achieve such effects as: a reduction in the intake of fats and cholesterol, a diminution in the use of tobacco and illicit drugs, the curtailment of drunk driving, and, in general, the adoption of health lifestyles (see Rice & Atkin, 1989; Rogers & Storey, 1987; Salmon, 1989). Without question, the dual paradigms of "individualism" and "communication effects" have dominated empirical research in communication since the inception of programmatic research on communication and persuasion earlier this century (Delia, 1987; Gitlin, 1978).

Preoccupation with the paradigm of individualism has simultaneously resulted in a relative dearth of scholarship, in communication circles, on macrolevel considerations of the change process (McLeod & Blumler, 1987). This neglect of attention to systemic change is unfortunate, some scholars have observed, because of the inherent reciprocity that exists between systems and individuals, between macro- and microlevels of analysis (Kelman & Warwick, 1978). As a result, we know a great deal more

131

about the effects of health communication on individuals' cognitions, attitudes, and behaviors than on, for example, the determinants of that communication (i.e., the interplay of institutional influences that shapes the structure and function of organized systems of communication activities). In other words, the focus on communication effects has resulted in a virtually universal conceptualization of communication campaigns as independent rather than dependent variables, as producers rather than themselves products of social change (Salmon, 1991).

This chapter departs from tradition by focusing on the evolution, structure, and function, rather than the effects, of a national communications system. Specifically, this chapter employs the framework of general systems theory to describe and analyze the National AIDS Information and Education Program (NAIEP), an organization that was created in response to the growing AIDS epidemic and charged with educating "the general public" about HIV and AIDS. This chapter has three distinct purposes. First, it describes principles of general systems theory, in the abstract, as a potentially useful lens or frame for analyzing an organization and its output. Second, it provides a description of NAIEP in terms of the principles of systems theory discussed earlier. The point of this section is to show how NAIEP can be defined both as a system of production—an organization—as well as a system of influence—as the product or output of the organization. Finally, the theoretical framework described initially is reexamined in terms of the specifics of NAIEP described in the second section. This reexamination represents an assessment of "correspondence" between systems theory and empirical observations (Monge, 1982).

GENERAL SYSTEMS THEORY

Ludwig von Bertalanffy (1955), a theoretical biologist and pivotal figure in the genesis of systems theory, was an early critic of reductionism, the attempt to reduce biological, behavioral, and social sciences to the constructs and laws of physics. He advocated an alternative that he described as "perspectivism," an interdisciplinary convergence predicated upon the unifying principle of organization. Operating from this premise, he proposed that all disciplines could benefit from the development of a general systems theory that would provide a structural-functional framework for the study of organization. Although the concepts and models comprising this general systems theory emanated from the natural sciences, they were quickly embraced and adapted by social scientists in such disciplines as sociology, anthropology, psychology, political science, and communication.

In its most basic essence, a system is an assembly of related elements interacting to perform specific functions, defined by physical or conceptual boundaries, and existing in some environment.[1] Systems are comprised of subsystems, smaller, less complex assemblages of elements, and can themselves be components of metasystems, that is, larger, more complex assemblages of systems. A decision regarding what actually constitutes a system therefore depends entirely on the level of analysis of interest to some observer-analyst. For example, a biologist may choose to define a system in terms of some bodily function (e.g., digestion or respiration) of a single individual. In contrast, a sociologist may define a system as a collectivity of individuals, whose homeostasis is maintained through the interplay of legal, financial, and social subsystems. In the first case, the individual could be treated as a metasystem or as an environment, whereas in the second, the individual could be treated as a subsystem.

A system may exist as a planned, intentionally interrelated set of elements, or as the serendipitous outcome of external forces. In addition, a system may exist as an actual physical entity or, alternatively, only in the abstract as defined by some observer or analyst. Thus the terms *behavioral systems, administrative systems, communication systems,* or *developmental systems* may refer to highly managed, empirically observable groups of components, or to functional linkages among a set of disparate or logically defined elements said to constitute a system (Clarke, 1985; Winett, 1986).

Systems that actively interact with environments outside their boundaries are described as *open,* whereas those that are isolated, neither affecting nor affected by their environments, are referred to as *closed.* In general, open systems are more practical, realistic, and hence more viable representations of social phenomena, particularly in today's "global village" characterized by shared cultures, economies, and political structures. An open system is able to both adapt to and effect changes in environments by virtue of its interactive nature. That is, the open system absorbs input (personnel, material resources, ideas, normative pressure, and information), adapts to fluctuations in various social, political, or economic environments, and, through performing its specific function, generates output (typically a product or idea) into its environments, thereby altering them in the process. The open system receives feedback from the environment, which becomes input to be used in decisions regarding the need for maintenance or adaptation.

---

[1]The discussion of general systems theory contained herein represents a compilation of theories, insights, and conclusions advanced by several scholars, especially von Bertalanffy (1955), Parsons (1956), Gross (1965), Berrien (1968), Monge (1977), Bronfenbrenner (1979), and Clarke (1985).

At the heart of the systems notion is the interdependence of various components or subsystems: The units comprising the system operate in concert to achieve a common goal. This interdependence usually implies the presence of some centralized guidance subsystem responsible for providing direction and coordination of functions (Gross, 1965). A key role of system management involves anticipating and adapting to trends in relevant political, social, and economic environments. Environments that are considered "placid" place little in the way of demands for organizational adaptation. In contrast, "turbulent" environments, those characterized by flux and deepening interdependence with other systems, mandate frequent monitoring (solicitation of feedback) and adaptation (Emery & Trist, 1965; Terreberry, 1968).

In practice, it is certainly conceivable that a person hired to develop and manage, for example, a community-based smoking cessation program would not consciously plan to create a formal system or religiously translate theoretical precepts into public health tactics. Nevertheless, what might begin as a mere agglomeration of apparently unrelated organizational tasks would, over time, evolve into an interdependent system as part of an inherent systemic tendency towards homeostasis. To use a very simple example, the use of broadcast public service announcements (PSAs) promoting the availability of free brochures would necessitate the linking of two distinct information subsystems—broadcast and print—and two marketing subsystems—promotion and distribution. The linkage that ultimately would evolve might be the result of prudent strategic planning or the unfortunate lack of planning and subsequent crisis management. Similarly, a decision to employ and maintain tactics other than the PSA and brochure would be dependent on the activities of other systems, such as competing health-care providers, as well as fluctuations in health, financial, and political environments. Thus, the system's evolution would be strongly influenced by the structure and function of competing systems, the dynamism of relevant environments, and feedback regarding successes and failures along the way.

THE GENERAL SYSTEMS PERSPECTIVE
AS AN ANALYTIC FRAMEWORK

Monge (1977) has specified the conditions necessary for analyzing a communications phenomenon as an open system. These conditions include:

1. a description of the system's evolution,
2. an identification of the system's components,
3. specification of the internal structure and relations among subsystems,

4. determination of the system's processes,
5. stipulation of the system's environment, and
6. a description of inputs and outputs.

In the present context, we can further distinguish between two distinct ways of defining a system, one that emphasizes the structure and function of an organization actually producing communication as an output and a second that focuses on the communication output itself. The use of a systems perspective to analyze the former is well established in social science research. A pioneer in this application, Talcott Parsons (1956), has defined an *organization* as a system that, to attain its goals, "produces an identifiable something which can be utilized in some way by another system; that is, output of the organization is, for some other system, an input" (p. 65). Essential to a systems analysis of organizations, Parsons continued, is an understanding of the dominant values of the system. Values legitimize and prioritize organizational goals; hence, the underlying value structure must be identified before the organization as a whole can be understood.

Defining organizational *output* as a system in and of itself is less common; more typically, output would be defined as a discrete entity (e.g., a product or service). Yet in the context of health communication, the output of an organization charged with educating the public of some health hazard is likely to consist of a system of communication rather than discrete, uncoordinated units. In large measure, this reflects the emerging consensus that single modes of communication, particularly mass, are inadequate in and of themselves for inducing significant degrees of social change and must instead be integrated vertically with other communication subsystems (e.g., interpersonal and organizational) or horizontally with other social-change subsystems (e.g., power or technology) to be effective (Salmon, 1991). Bronfenbrenner (1979); McLeroy, Bibeau, Steckler, and Glanz (1988); Winett (1986); and Ray and Donohew (1990) have described "systems of influence" that correspond to organizational output designed to effect social- and individual-level change. Bronfenbrenner and McLeroy et al., in particular, draw on general systems theory to detail a set of nested systems, ranging from the microsystem, an individual's immediate setting, to exosystems and macrosystems, that is, larger, more complex and more distant environments (such as public policy or, ultimately, culture), that directly and indirectly exert influence on individual development. Adopting such a perspective, a public health organization's communication output would be organized in terms of several hierarchically ordered subsystems: mass communication; community-based programs; communication programs for the workplace, schools, and other organizational environments; interpersonal channels;

and a network of coordination among subsystems. Only by anchoring change efforts in multiple systems of environmental influence, according to this line of reasoning, could a health program realistically hope to induce large-scale, enduring change.

The principles of general systems theory and the categorization scheme of system characteristics developed by Monge provide a useful lens for analyzing the structure and function of health organizations. In the next section, we use these frameworks to describe the evolution of NAIEP, first as an organizational system and second as a system of influence.

Evolution of NAIEP as an Organizational System

The public health communications system extant in the early 1980s was judged to be generally inadequate for the job of educating and stemming the anxieties of individuals and organizations confronting the disease firsthand. Between June 1981, when the first case reports of AIDS were published (Centers for Disease Control, 1981), and September 1987, when the Centers for Disease Control (CDC) launched the first phase of its national media campaign, there were no nationally coordinated efforts to educate the American people about the disease or ways to avoid infection (Kinsella, 1989). Instead, information was disseminated through the independent efforts of several social institutions and organizations, including the news media; a loosely knit array of community-based organizations, especially in such heavily impacted areas as New York City, San Francisco, and Los Angeles; and some components of the public health system, also mainly in heavily impacted areas of the country (Kroger, 1989).

In June 1986, the Public Health Service (PHS) summoned its top AIDS officials to Coolfont, West Virginia, which resulted in a brief report on a "PHS Plan for Prevention and Control of AIDS and the AIDS Virus" (Public Health Service, 1986). This report called for mass information-education programs directed toward the "currently uninfected population," infected persons, and other "individuals and groups whose behavior placed them at high risk for AIDS." Although the report's architects did not specifically use the terminology of communication systems, they did call for a multitiered, multidisciplinary set of educational initiatives that would draw on existing media and organizational channels to reach the diverse audiences in need of timely information, education, training, and counseling.

Concurrently, the Institute of Medicine (1986) published a comprehensive report entitled "Confronting AIDS: Directions for Public Health, Health Care, and Research," in which it criticized the federal AIDS education effort as "woefully inadequate." That year, the Department of

Health and Human Services had budgeted $120,000 for AIDS education (Kinsella, 1989). As a remedy, it called for a major educational campaign "to reduce the spread of HIV," and the establishment of a new office, possibly within the Office of the Assistant Secretary for Health, to implement and assess a massive, coordinated educational program.

In October 1986, Surgeon General Dr. C. Everett Koop (1986) released his "Report on Acquired Immune Deficiency." The report, as well as the person, helped to galvanize the public policy environment and generate support for the development of a federally funded AIDS communications system. Shortly thereafter, the PHS (1987) adopted and published a more detailed plan. This plan became the legislative blueprint for establishing an organization charged with the responsibility of educating "the public." In addition, it appropriated funds to support comprehensive school education programs, education and training programs for health-care workers, and expanded programs to reach individuals at high risk of infection. The implicit systems philosophy undergirding this proposal is shown in Fig. 7.1, excerpted from the PHS Plan, which demonstrates the extent to which the proposed communications system would have to work in concert with a variety of other national health and communications systems.

Congress assigned lead responsibility for prevention education to CDC which, in turn, established a new Program Office within the Director's Office of CDC. This decision regarding the placement of the Program Office was the result of an organizational belief that it was important to provide a high degree of internal visibility and support if the program was to succeed. It also imposed an uncommon level of review, oversight, and clearance for materials and activities, which at one time included review by the White House Domestic Policy Council. This degree of oversight was indicative of the extent to which the AIDS environment was highly politicized.

The internal organizational system of NAIEP was designed primarily in functional terms. That is, three subsystems were created to convert inputs of human and financial resources into outputs in the form of four types of communication believed to be important for a national information program. First, a media subsystem was established to develop, in conjunction with a national advertising agency, public service announcements for television, radio, magazines, newspapers, and auxiliary media such as billboards and transit. In addition, this subsystem was made responsible for generating news media coverage through the use of video news releases and press conferences.

A second subsystem was established primarily to coordinate a National AIDS Hotline (NAH) and National AIDS Clearinghouse (NAC). The NAH had been established in early 1983, and was originally staffed by public

138   SALMON AND KROGER

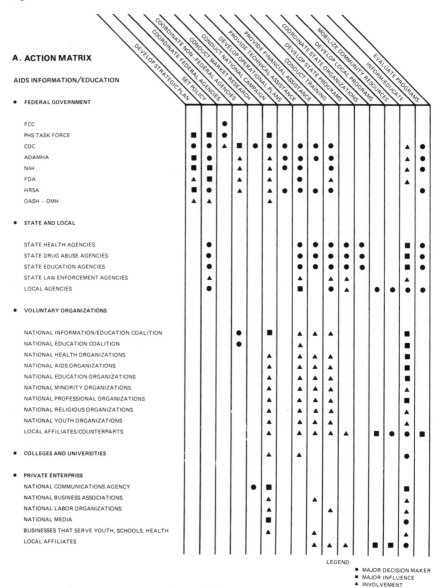

FIG. 7.1.   Action matrix from the PHS plan.

affairs personnel from various PHS agencies before being transferred to the CDC in 1985. The NAH, a type of "mass-interpersonal" communication, was designed to provide personal information services and referrals to health and social services, and to place orders for written materials. In 1988, NAH information specialists handled more than 2.2 million calls—the largest number of phone calls that any publicly funded health information telephone service had ever managed. The NAC was established in 1988 and, like NAH, has become the largest such system in U.S. public health history. In its first 3 years of operation, NAC distributed more than 60 million pieces of AIDS-related literature, primarily to health service organizations and individuals. In addition, the NAC manages several databases that include information on more than 14,000 services being provided by organizations throughout the United States, educational materials and programs developed for various target populations, and information about drug treatment trials and their protocols.

A third organizational subsystem was established to develop interpersonal, organizational, and community-level dimensions of the Program. This unit works with such organizations as the American Red Cross, the National AIDS Leadership Coalition, National Association of Persons with AIDS, the National Council of LaRaza, National Parents and Teachers Association, and the National Urban League in planning programs and disseminating materials.

The three subsystems work toward a common goal (i.e., enhancing the U.S. population's awareness of and knowledge about HIV and AIDS). The values underlying this goal are the product of multiple influences on NAIEP. Because it is a not-for-profit public health agency situated in the PHS, NAIEP is first of all concerned with promoting the public interest, health, and general welfare of citizens. Second, because it is a component of the CDC, which has been designated as the nation's prevention agency, NAIEP endorses the value of health maintenance through disease prevention. Third, NAIEP's value system is influenced by the value system of the medical profession, rooted in the Hippocratic Oath, which posits that a person responsible for health care should "do no harm." These organizational values represent alternative dimensions of the overarching value of serving the public interest; as such, they can result in conflicting implications for public policy. For example, in order to be in compliance with the value of "doing no harm," NAIEP has chosen to refrain from the use of heavy fear appeals in its public service announcements (which, some believe, might induce psychological harm). This observation is important for several reasons. First, it demonstrates how an organization translates an abstract value such as "harm" into a concrete campaign decision. Second, it reveals some of management's implicit assumptions about communication, health, and the public interest. That is, management assumes that communication is capable of inducing effects; that fear appeals will be ineffective or, even worse, induce boomerang effects that will be harmful to individuals and society; that the medical value of "doing no harm" refers to psychological (as well as physical) harm; and that this type of harm is a greater threat to the public interest than the harm that might result from the decision not to deploy the more aggressive tactics of heavy fear appeals.

Evolution of NAIEP as a System of Influence

The inherent difficulties associated with quickly constructing a large-scale communications program, yet operating with constraints endemic to government-sponsored programs, initially afforded scarce opportunities for NAIEP's communication output to function as a system per se. Organizational subsystems had been established and were beginning to engage in a variety of communications tasks. These included: developing TV, radio, and print public service announcements; quadrupling the capacity of the toll-free hotline; developing several grant programs for national organizations; and conducting public forums and meetings in 30 cities during October, designated by Congress as "AIDS Awareness and Prevention Month." Because of political pressures, as well as the overall sense of urgency motivating programmatic efforts, the initial phase of the "America Responds to AIDS" media campaign, the organizational output made possible by a financial input of $21 million in public funds, was largely national in scope and designed predominantly to heighten public awareness of and sensitivity to AIDS.

Outside of NAIEP, school health programs, clinic-based counseling and testing programs, outreach efforts for drug users, national, state and local communications programs, and financial assistance programs to racial and ethnic minority organizations were being developed concurrently, but often by different organizational systems within PHS. No common blueprints existed to govern and coordinate the content, quality, or principal foci of the diverse programs.

A major turning point in converting this set of nonintegrated activities into an integrated system of influence was the development and distribution of the national household mailer, *Understanding AIDS,* which constituted the second phase of the national campaign. Because the mailer represented a public health activity of unprecedented scope, it required a heretofore absent degree of coordination among systems and subsystems alike. First, senior officials throughout the CDC and PHS had to agree on the content of the brochure, particularly with regard to information concerning risk behaviors, the blood supply, and condom efficacy. Next, because the brochure was expected to generate phone calls to national, state, and local hotlines and to increase requests for HIV testing, information networks and clinic services needed advance warning to prepare for such events. Further, draft copies of the mailer were shared with public and private health officials, major AIDS service organizations, and the news media to ensure that the public would be alerted to the content, nature, and purpose of the mailing before it arrived. For the first time since the first cases of AIDS had been reported, virtually all communication and public health systems and subsystems dealing with AIDS were mobilized to speak with a clear, consistent voice on how the disease is and is not transmitted.

One hundred seven million copies of the mailer, which was explicit about such subjects as condoms and anal intercourse, were delivered to every household in the United States and its territories, and an additional 10 million copies were distributed to homeless shelters, correctional institutions, military installations, and to Foreign Service and Peace Corps personnel overseas. The mailer was the most widely read publication in the United States during June and July 1988 (Davis, 1991). The NAH as well as some local hotlines handled record numbers of calls. In addition, the NAC received requests from individuals and organizations for millions of additional copies of the mailer and for other informational items. Finally, the mailout contributed directly to the permanent addition of hotline services for Spanish-speaking and deaf audiences.

The system of influence forged of necessity in 1988 has continued to evolve and incrementally increase in complexity. The third phase of NAIEP's campaign was launched in October 1988, targeting women at risk and multiple partner, sexually active adults. The NAC and NAH conducted special training programs and database expansions to allow women at risk, who might need social support as a consequence of the campaign's message of empowerment, to obtain appropriate referrals.

The fourth phase of the campaign, targeting parents and youth, included several national partners, especially those involved with youth education. For the first time, state health departments were also incorporated into plans for information distribution. In October 1988, state AIDS program leaders assembled in Dallas, Texas, for the first AIDS communications conference in an effort to improve the public health community's capacity to implement the national campaign.

The fifth phase of the campaign, "Preventing HIV Infection and AIDS: Taking the Next Steps," marked the involvement of multicultural consultants drawn from the CDC's minority grant recipients to assure cultural appropriateness of campaign materials for African-American and Hispanic audiences. To assist local health departments gain greater public service time and news coverage for AIDS, the program conducted community workshops in 15 cities for which Broadcast Advertisers Report (BAR) data reflected lower-than-average public service attention to AIDS. Assisted by the National Association of Broadcasters, the workshops brought news and public service directors from local media outlets together with national, state, and local public health officials for the purpose of establishing contacts and cultivating ongoing relationships.

Currently, NAIEP is one of several systems operating within the CDC charged with the responsibility of HIV prevention. Its annual operating budget of approximately $25 million represents about 5% of CDC's budget for HIV-AIDS, and less than 2% of the total Public Health Service expenditures for HIV-AIDS in fiscal 1991 (Noble, Parra, & Holman, 1991). NAIEP's efforts to educate "the public" thus do not occur in a vacuum; they operate in conjunction with other CDC organizations, such as the National Center for Chronic Disease Prevention and Health Promotion, which coordinates school education, minority outreach programs and behavioral surveillance; the National Center for Prevention Services, which coordinates state and local HIV prevention efforts and risk-reduction programs; and the National Institute for Occupational Health and Safety, which is responsible for issues involving HIV in the workplace.

Discussion

The systems perspective has been offered as a frame through which a communications organization, NAIEP, can be described and analyzed. NAIEP was forged through the interaction of a host of political, economic, social, and medical influences; however, it, like virtually all programs of its kind, was not influenced by a conscious application of an academic theory, which is being applied in this analysis post hoc. Thus, lack of convergence between theory and empiricism should not be interpreted as failure of the organization to adhere to theoretical principles, but instead, failure of the theory to explain the particular. Given this caveat, there are several important points to be made about NAIEP as a system.

First, as Monge (1977) has observed, social and communication systems do not have a fixed, inherent structure, but instead "create themselves in response to the challenge of the environment." This has certainly been the case with NAIEP to date. The AIDS environment is an especially challenging one, characterized by rancorous policy debates, a multitude of conflicting interests seeking representation in programmatic decisions, changing needs of the public, unpredictable reports of potentially life-threatening situations fueling public concern, and uncertainties regarding the development of noncommunication alternatives to HIV prevention, such as vaccines. As such, the AIDS environment is best characterized in the terms of Emery and Trist (1965) as a "turbulent field," a high degree of uncertainty and a deepening interdependence in legislation and public regulation.

The organizational structure that NAIEP initially adopted—designed in terms of communication functions—represented a response to the environment at the time: The organization was founded a full 6 years after cases of AIDS were first reported, and was expected to very quickly supply information to a public that was perceived as needy. The sense of urgency that served as the impetus for the initial structure has not abated in the face of an unflinchingly turbulent environment; it is reinforced regularly with every highly publicized case involving HIV and AIDS. Maintained throughout the shifting and settling of environments are the organization's primary values of health promotion and the avoidance of harm. At times, these values can conflict, as any communication activity, to paraphrase Bernard Berelson's famous aphorism, may have an adverse effect on some persons under some conditions. In such situations, a balancing of organizational values occurs and a communications product is produced that is compatible with the value systems.

As a way of coping with the demands of a turbulent environment, NAIEP has maintained a version of an open systems philosophy, operationalized through frequent meetings with representatives of other, interested systems, constant monitoring of research and popular publications, and primary data collection in the form of focus groups, field experiments, and national surveys. Although an informal feedback mechanism was instituted concurrently with the inception of the program, a formal subsystem devoted to feedback was not added until 2 years later (Salmon & Jason, 1991). The combination of formal and informal feedback mechanisms at least creates the potential for the organization to successfully adapt to environmental fluctuations.

The notion of adaptation and change is critical to an understanding of the open systems concept, as well as the system at hand. NAIEP has become increasingly complex as it has evolved into a system of influence, developing targeted campaigns, integrating the efforts of state health departments, coordinating national conferences, and conducting media-advocacy workshops. In addition, its campaign themes have diversified over time from initial warnings about HIV transmission to more recent portrayals of persons living with AIDS. These changes in organizational functions and communication output reflect adaptation as well as conscious efforts to change. Theories of organizational change can be classified in terms of three types of precipitating causes: purposeful action, necessity, and chance (Aldrich & Marsden, 1988; Corning, 1983). In general, the evolution of NAIEP is best explained by a hybrid of a theory of necessity and secondarily by a theory of purposeful action. That is, the majority of major changes in organizational structure and function have been rooted in necessity (i.e., in response to external social, political, economic, and administrative pressures and, particularly in the initial stages, from lack of coordination among subsystems). As a governmental agency subject to the multitude of often-conflicting agendas, interests, and values inherent in a pluralistic political culture, NAIEP has operated largely in a reactive rather than proactive mode, and has been constrained in its use of terminology, images, and recommendations in its message appeals.

CONCLUSION

As Talcott Parsons (1961) argued, the study of structure is logically prior to an understanding of structural change. In general, Parsons' advice has not been heeded in scholarship on communication campaigns and information programs. With few exceptions, reviews of the campaign literature have attempted to draw sweeping generalizations about campaign effectiveness across a multitude of topics, settings, and audiences without taking into account key situational variables such as the structure and function of a given information program. Instead, campaigns and programs have been treated as rather homogeneous independent variables instead of quite heterogeneous dependent variables in their own right. This results in conclusions that are ambiguous scientifically and of questionable generalizability in the realm of public policy.

Whatever happens in society regarding individuals' knowledge of, attitudes toward, and behavior regarding HIV and AIDS will, to some degree, be determined by the structure and functions of systems of influence organized to induce social change. NAIEP is only one of a number of such systems, although it is certainly the most extensive and complex. By understanding the system, its genesis, its politicized constraints, and its role in the metasystem of the Public Health Service, we will have a better context in which to evaluate NAIEP's impact at the individual level of analysis, as well as to understand the more general process of social change that occurs at the macrolevel of analysis.

ACKNOWLEDGMENTS

Much of the work for this chapter was completed while Charles Salmon was a visiting communications researcher with the Centers for Disease Control.

The authors would like to thank Paul Farnham, Janine Jason, Beverly Schwartz, and Dianne Rucinski for their helpful comments on an earlier draft.

REFERENCES

Aldrich, H. E., & Marsden, P. V. (1988). Environments and organizations. In N. J. Smelser (Ed.), *Handbook of sociology* (pp. 361–392). Newbury Park, CA: Sage.

Berrien, F. K. (1968). *General and social systems.* New Brunswick, NJ: Rutgers University Press.

Bronfenbrenner, U. (1979). *The ecology of human development: Experiments by nature and design.* Cambridge, MA: Harvard University Press.

Centers for Disease Control. (1981, June 5). Pneumocystis pneumonia—Los Angeles. *Morbidity and Mortality Weekly Report, 30,* 250–252.

Clarke, D. D. (1985). *Action systems: An introduction to the analysis of complex behaviour.* London: Methuen.

Corning, P. A. (1983). *The synergism hypothesis.* New York: McGraw-Hill.

Davis, D. (1991). Understanding AIDS—The national AIDS mailer. *Public Health Reports, 106*(6), 656–662.

Delia, J. G. (1987). Communication research: A history. In C. R. Berger & S. H. Chaffee (Eds.), *Handbook of communication science* (pp. 20–98). Newbury Park, CA: Sage.

Emery, J. E., & Trist, E. L. (1965). The causal texture of organizational environments. *Human Relations, 18,* 21–32.

Gitlin, T. (1978). Media sociology: The dominant paradigm. *Theory and Society, 6,* 205–253.

Gross, B. A. (1965). What are your organization's objectives? A general-systems approach to planning. *Human Relations, 18,* 195–216.

Institute of Medicine. (1986). *Confronting AIDS: Directions for public health, health care, and research.* Washington, DC: National Academy Press.

Kelman, H. C., & Warwick, D. P. (1978). Bridging micro and macro approaches to social change: A social-psychological perspective. In G. Zaltman (Ed.), *Processes and phenomena of social change* (pp. 13–59). Huntington, NY: Krieger.

Kinsella, J. (1989). *Covering the plague: AIDS and the American media.* New Brunswick, NJ: Rutgers University Press.

Koop, C. E. (1986). *Surgeon General's report on Acquired Immune Deficiency Syndrome.* Washington, DC: U.S. Department of Health and Human Services.

Kroger, F. (1989, January). *Risk communication: HIV infection.* Paper presented at the American Association for the Advancement of Science, San Francisco.

McLeod, J. M., & Blumler, J. G. (1987). The macrosocial level of communication science. In C. R. Berger & S. H. Chaffee (Eds.), *Handbook of communication science* (pp. 271–322). Newbury Park, CA: Sage.

McLeroy, K. R., Bibeau, D., Steckler, A., & Glanz, K. (1988). An ecological perspective on health promotion programs. *Health Education Quarterly, 15,* 351–377.

Monge, P. R. (1977). The systems perspective as a theoretical basis for the study of human communication. *Communication Quarterly, 25,* 19–29.

Monge, P. R. (1982). Systems theory and research in the study of organizational communication: The correspondence problem. *Human Communication Research, 8,* 245–261.

Noble, G., Parra, W. C., & Holman, P. B. (1991). Organizational structure and resources of CDC's HIV-AIDS prevention program. *Public Health Reports, 106*(6), 604–607.

Parsons, T. (1956). Suggestions for a sociological approach to the theory of organizations—I. *Administrative Science Quarterly, 1,* 63–85.

Parsons, T. (1961). Some considerations on the theory of social change. *Rural Sociology, 26,* 219–239.

Public Health Service. (1986). The Coolfont report: Public health service plan for combatting AIDS. *Public Health Reports, 101,* 341–348.

Public Health Service. (1987). *Information/education plan to prevent and control AIDS in the United States.* Washington, DC: Author.

Ray, E. B., & Donohew, L. (Eds.). (1990). *Communication and health: Systems and applications.* Hillsdale, NJ: Lawrence Erlbaum Associates.

Rice, R., & Atkin, C. (Eds.). (1989). *Public communication campaigns.* Newbury Park, CA: Sage.

Rogers, E. M., & Storey, J. D. (1987). Communication campaigns. In C. R. Berger & S. H. Chaffee (Eds.), *Handbook of communication science* (pp. 817–846). Newbury Park, CA: Sage.

Salmon, C. T. (Ed.). (1989). *Information campaigns: Balancing social values and social change.* Newbury Park, CA: Sage.

Salmon, C. T. (1991). Bridging theory "of" and theory "for" communication campaigns: An essay on ideology and public policy. In S. Deetz (Ed.), *Communication yearbook 15* (pp. 346–358). Newbury Park, CA: Sage.

Salmon, C. T., & Jason, J. (1991). A system for evaluating the use of media in CDC's national AIDS information and education program. *Public Health Reports, 106*(6), 639–645.

Terreberry, S. (1968). The evolution of organizational environments. *Administrative Science Quarterly, 12,* 590–613.

von Bertalanffy, L. (1955). General systems theory. In N. J. Demerath, III & R. A. Peterson (Eds.), *System, change, and conflict* (pp. 115–129). New York: The Free Press.

Winett, R. A. (1986). *Information and behavior: Systems of influence.* Hillsdale, NJ: Lawrence Erlbaum Associates.

CHAPTER EIGHT

The Place of Culture in HIV Education

Paula Michal-Johnson
Sheryl Perlmutter Bowen
Villanova University

There is incontrovertible evidence that HIV has a far more profound effect in communities of color and in the gay community than in any others in the United States. Although Blacks constitute about 12% of the population and Latinos comprise 7%, 27% of people with AIDS are Black and 15% are Latino (Bowles & Robinson, 1989). Although early cases of AIDS were predominantly in men, rates of infection among women of color have risen drastically. In 1989 it was one of the 10 leading causes of death in women of reproductive age, and it may soon be one of the top five causes of death for women of color, if current projections hold (Chu, Buehler, & Berkelman, 1990). These disturbing figures help to clarify how HIV has intruded on the lives of individuals with differing cultural experiences.

HIV education and prevention efforts that take into account the cultural experiences of those who bear the disproportionate burden of AIDS have the best opportunity to offer believable messages and messengers in communities of color. We have five goals in writing this chapter. They are to: (a) define HIV education as a cultural communication process, (b) identify the models of culture used in HIV education, (c) explore the adequacy of health behavior-change models in mapping cultural communication processes, (d) assess the adequacy and relevance of intercultural literature in describing and explaining HIV education for individuals with different cultural experiences, and finally, (e) describe the tools researchers currently use to access the cultural communication process inherent in HIV education.

HIV EDUCATION AS A CULTURAL COMMUNICATION PROCESS

We argue that culture should be a central organizing concept in developing programs of HIV education and assessing their outcomes. Currently there are multicultural HIV education programs in all major metropolitan centers that address the concerns of gay men, African-Americans, Latinos, and IV drug users (IVDUs). The extent of multiculturalism required by HIV education is affected by the degree of association that individuals who engage in high-risk behaviors maintain with their cultural communities of origin. Essentially, those who remain in their own communities have culturally driven networks tied to a particular cultural orientation. Those who move out of their own communities interact within a multicultural framework. So at-risk individuals may meet in gay bars or bookstores, in shooting galleries, in low-income public housing projects, in shelters for the homeless, in drug rehabilitation programs, as well as work or social sites. Education targeted to people in any of these sites requires sensitivity to the cultural elements that influence the interactions taking place there.

We think of culture as a dynamic, multicomponent process. For instance, the cultural norms defining gender roles, language use, the willingness of partners to talk about sex, as well as partners' social and economic lives, all affect the process of safer-sex negotiation. When we choose to understand those culturally influenced communicative behaviors relevant in performing particular practices, we are looking at a series of phenomena in a dynamic environment. We call this intermeshing of living cultural imprints with the communication process the *cultural communication process.* This process is affected by race, ethnicity, social class, history, economic status, and gender. Culture is not viewed simply as one variable or even a set of variables, differentiating one group from another. Culture is a set of meanings and practices that are highly contextualized, not only by situation but also by historical context.

Culture is performed through human symbolic activity (Geertz, 1973; Mumby, 1989; Schneider, 1976; Turner, 1974). Culture is thus *enacted* by social actors. Servaes (1989) defined *cultures* as "social settings in which a certain reference framework has taken concrete form or has been institutionalized and orients and structures the interaction and communication of people within this historical context" (p. 390). Thus, in educating an African-American sex worker[1] who supports a drug habit, the HIV educator needs to understand the cultural communication process as it works for her. How she communicates with her customers, what she values in customers, how she relates to health information, her attitudes about her life, and her relationships with her children are all important conditions in her life. Gathering the detailed personal/cultural schema for each person receiving HIV education is not feasible. Consequently, the HIV educator will want to understand the patterned ways that sex workers adjust to their work, knowing how they communicate with clients, when they are least likely to use protection, and further, to understand the drug culture that often is connected with them.

Culture as a construct does not presume homogeneity in labels like African-American, Latino, Asian, Italian American, or other standard categories of race or ethnicity in the United States. As interpreted in this chapter, culture is not viewed as a monolithic term. Rather there are many variations on the underlying theme of culture. An individual might be a working-class African-American male living in a multicultural Spanish-speaking neighborhood. It is extremely difficult to identify the separate influence of each of these cultural elements. The term *culture,* then, collapses what others see as "demographic" variables, such as age, race, religion, ethnic heritage, socioeconomic class, and gender into one constellation, that for each individual would be somewhat idiosyncratic. The task each HIV educator faces is judging correctly which aspects of the cultural communication process are most relevant for group members in an educational setting at a particular time.

Those who study culture often use a "lens" metaphor to describe how individual members of a culture "see" the world. The lens, then, functions as the sum total of their experience projected onto any situation. In thinking about HIV education and cultural communication processes, the lens analogy breaks down. Instead, the educator in different cultural environments is faced with a need to understand the apparent cultural frameworks of the audiences, as well as the host of factors described previously. Perhaps a more complete metaphor for HIV educators incorporates a series of layers of transparency films that, when illuminated, produce a particular, composite color. In each different setting for HIV education the educator would "see" a different gestalt/hue. To promote behavioral change, education must address the cultural process in a believable and reasonable context, if there is hope of reaching the hardest to reach by tapping into how cultural communication processes operate.

The following sections seek to explicate the extent to which HIV edu-

---

[1]The term *sex worker* is used here rather than prostitute or other terms that have negative connotations.

cation in the United States and models of health behavior change accommodate cultural communication processes. In some we see culture in sharp focus, in others it fades into the background.

CULTURAL CONTEXTS FOR PROVIDING HIV EDUCATION

With this definition of cultural communication processes in mind, we explore how it has been operationalized in AIDS/HIV education in the United States. Essentially there are two primary avenues for AIDS education: public health providers and community-based organizations. Each approach signals differing levels of commitment to designing culturally compatible education. The following discussion assumes that programs may function on a continuum of sorts ranging from culture-free, to culturally adapted, to culture-specific.

In generic education the Centers for Disease Control (CDC; 1988) offers what might be considered culture-free advice about how to conduct AIDS education. For example, guidelines encourage age-appropriate instruction and techniques that will promote role-playing and involvement, with little concern for cultural issues. Approaches like this encourage thinking of all 15-year-olds as fundamentally the same. Former Surgeon General C. Everett Koop's mailed pamphlet represents this approach.

Where it is possible for public institutions serving multicultural communities, culture may be considered from the cultural adaptation point of view. This incorporates culture as descriptive of the audience and espouses message design that accommodates the primary cultural attitudes, values, beliefs, and practices of diverse members of a community.

One strategy using the cultural adaptation model to implement a more sensitive program requires cultural input from minority leaders in the formulation of HIV educational campaigns. The National Minority AIDS Council has influenced the policies and services of the CDC and National Institutes for Health. The CDC has enhanced its access to African-American and Latino community AIDS educators through networks and review panels. Likewise, the American Red Cross has undertaken an extensive project assigning African-American Red Cross employees and volunteers to create a training manual to sensitize Red Cross trainers to the cultural issues and cultural styles specific to African-American youth. The American Red Cross manual (1990) was produced in concert with the National Urban League, and leaders in African-American HIV education positions reviewed the manual for accuracy and appropriateness. The cultural adaptation model reinforces the conclusion that regardless of whether the AIDS educator is culturally similar to the target audience, he or she must be able to conceptualize the curriculum from the values and experiences of the intended audience. In presenting, the educator must use a verbal style that the audience will find believable and persuasive. However, constructing the strategies for each specific curriculum requires an identification with those elements of lived experience that are "normal" and part of everyday events. It is difficult to argue that one can learn all there is to know about the workings of a culture without the inherent imprint of that culture on the psyche, hence the culture-specific model may be a preferred orientation to HIV education when education involves only members of one primary culture.

Culture-specific AIDS education approaches culture as the core unifying element that defines HIV education. This model suggests that only those who can effectively model the culture, understanding its subtleties, can legitimately conduct HIV education. Culture-specific education relies on the supposition that cultural similarity is crucial to the intervention. It is clear that one of the major barriers to providing effective education is "how" the information is delivered and by whom. As De La Cancela (1989) noted, "many Blacks and Latinos will be likely to listen more carefully to a prevention message emanating from people of color than they will to one from White, male, middle class authorities or even government officials" (p. 146).

Culture-specific education seems mandatory when the African-American experience with AIDS is studied. Although individual African-Americans were affected by HIV in the early 1980s, the larger African-American community denied existence of the disease and delayed prevention efforts. Dalton (1989) explained the slow acceptance of the health risks of HIV by members of the Black community through at least five factors:

1. a sense of blaming of African-Americans for bringing the disease to America,
2. a deep-seated suspicion and mistrust many Blacks felt when Whites expressed a sudden interest in them,
3. homophobia within the Black community that promoted denial of homosexuality and bisexuality,
4. the phenomenon of drug abuse in the Black community, and
5. tremendous resentment at being dictated to.

The reasons for this slow acceptance of the epidemiology are thus tied to common historical/cultural experiences within the Black community.

It is possible to see each of these three cultural perspectives in use within a given agency, based on the goals of the program. Consider the task of public health providers whose institutions are committed to serving the entire population within its geographic locale. This means that health-care providers connected to national, state, regional, or city health services are mandated to serve individuals of many cultures. In addition, organizations like the American Red Cross, hospitals, and private clinics may offer HIV education to the extent that it serves their interests. These public access educational efforts may offer information on site only or provide community education. In Philadelphia's Sexually Transmitted Disease (STD) Clinic, on-site education is the norm. For the most part, the clinic assists African-American and Latino men diagnosed with syphilis or gonorrhea. All clinic attenders view videos designed for Black clientele in the waiting room prior to examination and while they wait for test results. The soap opera videos designed for the CDC by Solomon and DeJong (1986) are specifically targeted to inner-city Black men. In this clinic, cultural adaptation has occurred in the videos. However, health-care providers conducting patient education may not themselves be culturally similar to those seeking services. Interviews with STD clinic physicians and educators suggest extreme variability in levels of sensitivity to current clients (Michal-Johnson, 1988).

Thus, culturally adapted tools can be integrated into a system alongside culture-free education. The three different strategies: culture-free, cultural adaptation, and culture-specific HIV education also illustrate the extent to which culture should be seen as a primary influencing process. Ideally we would advocate culture-specific education in most instances, but realize that health communities may have to settle for culturally adapted education.

THE RELEVANCE OF CULTURE
AND COMMUNICATION IN MODELS
OF HEALTH BEHAVIOR CHANGE

Academicians attempt to understand why some people adopt preventive behaviors and others do not, whereas those who design interventions try to predict which message and program strategies will be most effective in yielding desired behavioral changes. Because many programs were developed with a primary concern of diminishing the spread of HIV infection, it took some time before theoretical models that had been applied to other health behaviors such as immunization and smoking cessation, were applied to AIDS. The three primary models used in attempts to understand AIDS-related health attitudes and behaviors are Fishbein and Ajzen's Theory of Reasoned Action (Fishbein & Middlestadt, 1989), Becker et al.'s Health Behavior Model (Becker & Joseph, 1988; Kirscht

& Joseph, 1989), and Bandura's Social-Cognitive Theory of Self-Efficacy (Bandura, 1990). Our purpose here is not to provide an extensive review of each of the models, but rather to explore how the concepts of culture and communication have been included in each of these perspectives. We also review how concepts from the models have been used in empirical studies of AIDS-related behaviors in an effort to further our understanding of AIDS education as a cultural communication process.

Theory of Reasoned Action

Fishbein and Middlestadt (1989) utilized Ajzen and Fishbein's (1980) Theory of Reasoned Action (TRA) to explore AIDS-related behaviors. TRA is the most highly refined of the three models in terms of specifying the relationships among the theoretical variables. "In some respects, the theory is best looked at as a series of hypotheses linking (a) behavior to intentions, (b) intentions to a weighted combination of attitudes and subjective norms, and (c) attitudes and subjective norms to behavioral and normative beliefs, respectively" (Fishbein & Middlestadt, 1989, p. 95). In their essay, as in other essays that elaborate the theory, Fishbein and Middlestadt are careful to note the cultural relativity of attitudes, perceived norms of one's reference groups, beliefs about the outcomes of behaviors, and beliefs about the behaviors of one's normative group. They provide many examples, some considering Black and Latino men, and suggest that to change behavior, one must target the relevant components of the model with the greatest influence on behavioral intent. From this perspective, prior research is necessary to discover the salient target behaviors and beliefs. There does seem to be some evidence that the importance of culture is presumed, but only as culture influences one's attitudes and beliefs about specific actions. Programs utilizing this framework might thus be characterized in the cultural adaptation area of the continuum discussed earlier. This model also emphasizes a highly rational decision-making process, a presumption that may not be entirely relevant for AIDS-related behaviors that are heavily influenced by emotions. Careful attention to audience selection is crucial for effective campaigns, and indeed, for results that will support the theory of reasoned action.

Communication per se is thus not an integral part of TRA, but inferentially, it is not inconsistent with the model. Communication can be the outcome of a reasoned decision, for example, an expressed intention to perform a particular behavior, such as using a condom the next time the individual has sex, or talking about AIDS prevention with one's potential sex partner. Pre- and posttests can assess whether beliefs or attitudes change through a particular communicative strategy such as media messages or peer support.

Health Belief Model

The Health Belief Model (HBM), admittedly, was developed to explain much less severe health threats, such as immunizations or dietary changes (Becker, 1974; Janz & Becker, 1984; Rosenstock, 1974). The HBM details four essential components to explain why an individual is likely to change a particular action: personal susceptibility, perceived severity, the value (benefits, efficacy, or effectiveness) of a behavior, and barriers to the action (Kirscht & Joseph, 1989). Cultural and demographic variables are seen as exogenous. Witte (in press) noted that in the HBM, as in other treatments of persuasion, cultural variables are relevant as peripheral cues, not directly tied in the mind of the actor to the particular action. These peripheral cues, such as similarity between communicator and target audience in terms of cultural identification, language, and credibility, can affect choices for the message source. Receiver variables, such as education, also affect the persuasive process but only in an indirect way. We would argue that every aspect of the persuasive process is imbued with culture, and that cultural influences must be recognized in the process of developing effective campaigns discouraging AIDS risk behaviors. Programs demonstrating cultural specificity would not be expected out of this model.

Communication, in some treatments of HBM, is a cue to action, one that might get a person to change attitude or behavior. We would suggest that communication is integral to the process of change. One perceives the severity or susceptibility of the disease often as a result of communication. The communication may take the shape of a mediated message such as a public service announcement (PSA), or in today's culture, a talk show, like the Oprah Winfrey show. Interpersonal communication with peers or respected sources may also trigger a desired change in belief or attitude.

Numerous studies assess knowledge, attitudes, and behaviors relevant to AIDS using survey items that are derived from the HBM. Montgomery et al. (1989) found that the perceptions of the impact of the epidemic and the demands it places on individuals have greatly affected the perceptions of the severity of AIDS. These perceptions were linked to behavioral change in the Montgomery et al. study. In addition, socioeconomic advantage, barriers to change (including the stress involved with changing behaviors), and nonsupportive peer norms were also found to be related to the level of behavioral change. Susceptibility was not found to have a significant effect (also see Kirscht & Joseph, 1989).

In addition to the studies reviewed by Montgomery et al. (1989), many other researchers cited the HBM as informing the choice of questions asked on their surveys. For example, Koopman, Rotheram-Borus, Henderson, Bradley, and Hunter (1990) and Manning, Barenberg, Gallese, and Rice (1989) have reported studies with college students. The Health Belief Model, then, becomes a research tool with which correlations among variables are sought. The model is not often discussed in the literature as a plan for developing programs for AIDS-related behavior change.

Nyamathi and her colleagues (Flaskerud & Nyamathi, 1989; Flaskerud & Rush, 1989; Nyamathi & Shin, 1990; Nyamathi, Shuler, & Porche, 1990) provided a welcome exception to the dearth of program-related studies found in conjunction with the HBM. They are engaged in an ongoing project to provide AIDS education from Black and Latina women to Black and Latina women. Although results documenting effectiveness have not yet found their way into print, this project is remarkable in that it was theoretically motivated. The intervention was carefully designed using findings from extensive reviews of previous research and grounded research.

Nyamathi and Shin (1990) offered a cogent description of the parameters surrounding AIDS-related beliefs and practices for Black and Latina women. They discuss, for example, why women in these groups may be less likely to see themselves at risk (susceptibility), why many women who are poor and uneducated and have little medical knowledge may be unconcerned about AIDS (severity). They observe the numerous barriers that must be overcome to achieve behavior change, and argue that the benefits should be promoted through the existing ethic of social responsibility rather than individualistic preservation (also see Nyamathi et al., 1990). Their work is drawn both from the literature (e.g., work by Mays & Cochran, 1988) as well as from focus groups done with women from the communities they are attempting to serve (Flaskerud & Rush, 1989). This work demonstrates extreme sensitivity to the differences faced by Black women and by Latina women. Their questionnaire data show that Black women's knowledge is somewhat greater than the level of knowledge for Latina women, whereas sexual and drug practices are not significantly different between the groups (Flaskerud & Nyamathi, 1989). These findings suggest that messages to Black and Latina women cannot be identical.

Nyamathi ultimately offered guidelines for designing a culturally specific program for Black and Latina women. Psychological and cultural considerations suggest that the educational messages emanate from women who have backgrounds similar to the clients. Respect, trust, and empowerment must guide all intervention interactions. The education attempts to go beyond "AIDS 101" of transmission routes and epidemiology, in suggesting substitute activities that can be integrated into women's lifestyles without fear of negative judgment. Skills training, including work with communication skills for negotiating condom use and providing sex education for one's children, is also included. It is refreshing to see theoretical grounding providing an avenue for praxis in this culturally specific project.

Nonetheless, Nyamathi's work goes beyond the Health Belief Model, adding other variables to the pool. Indeed as Kirscht and Joseph (1989) summarized, the HBM "has useful features, but it requires synthesis with other frameworks for change" (p. 124).

Social Learning Theory and Self-Efficacy

Bandura, using the concept of self-efficacy as the force driving successful behavior change, clearly admitted the importance of culture and cultural variations in particular beliefs and practices. In outlining components of effective programs of self-directed change, Bandura (1990) argued that people need to be given reasons to alter risky habits and the means and resources to do so (p. 128). People first need information to increase awareness and knowledge. Next, they need to develop social and self-regulatory skills needed to translate information into preventive action. Third, the programs must be "aimed at skill enhancement and building resilient self-efficacy by providing opportunities for guided practice and corrective feedback in applying the skills in high-risk situation. The final component involves enlisting social supports for desired personal changes" (Bandura, 1990, p. 130). In providing a tailored educational message with an important modeling component, Bandura assumed intimate knowledge of the target audience, suggesting a culturally adaptive or culturally specific approach. He even advised that existing organizations that are relevant to community members be used for disseminating messages about AIDS prevention. Such organizations may be social, religious, recreational, occupational, or educational (p. 132).

Bandura's approach is thus more practical than the previous two approaches, and as a result, communication is central to attaining goals for an intervention or campaign. Maibach (1989) provided a schema for an AIDS prevention video message utilizing Bandura's principles. According to Maibach, in addition to teaching individuals how to perform the necessary skills for reducing risk, those who model the behaviors should be similar to the audience in gender, age, race, and attitudes. Safer-sex strategies should be demonstrated in settings similar to those that viewers will encounter. Brooks-Gunn, Boyer, and Hein (1988), and Flora and Thoresen (1988) also drew upon Bandura's work in studying adolescents and AIDS.

Solomon and DeJong (1986) conducted grounded research in an educational intervention project dealing with sexually transmitted infections.

Their work, which was also influenced by Bandura's theory, suggests that culture is a relevant construct in providing educational services. Specifically, they tell us that the health educator should: (a) explicitly discuss the precise circumstances under which the new behavior is to be carried out, the benefits of doing so, and the consequences of failing to do so; (b) acknowledge obstacles to change, build in supports and reinforcements for adopting new behaviors; and (c) promote identification between the client and the message. Each of these processes is deeply embedded in the socio/economic/cultural realities of the individual. It is first necessary to learn what life is like for an individual, how she or he sees the world, and the phenomena under study, before change can realistically take place as a result of preventive messages.

AIDS Risk-Reduction Model

Catania and his colleagues (see Catania et al., 1989; Catania, Gibson, Marin, Coates, & Greenblatt, 1990; Coates, 1990) have developed an AIDS risk-reduction model (ARRM) that uses elements of all three of the models—TRA, HBM, and self-efficacy—along with theories of help-seeking to explain preventive actions. The ARRM postulates three stages of the change process: labeling, commitment, and enactment. Communication here is an outcome variable, in the enactment stage, where individuals communicate with primary and new partners about risk reduction, they may network with others in their communities, and seek help from formal channels in sustaining the modified behaviors. Catania et al. (1989) limited their discussion to the gay male community, but noted that the approach may be used in community-based interventions among heterosexual, teen, adult, and minority populations (p. 258). Coates (1990) has argued that intervention research should be a priority in risk groups. Coates believes that information, motivational factors, skills training, and modifying perceived norms can be used for interventions. No evaluation studies were available at this time to support the claims of the ARRM's proponents.

General Accounting Office Model

Another model for the development of prevention messages has integrated many of the findings of previous efforts by social scientists and practitioners (Longshore, 1990). Derived inductively from interviews with experts who chose exemplary AIDS prevention programs, the General Accounting Office (GAO) model applies only to the development of prevention messages, and not to program development. This model is entirely germane to the communication process, and incorporates, at least broadly, sensitivity to cultural differences. At least the following seven factors should be considered, according to Longshore:

1. target group boundaries
2. characteristics placing the group at risk
3. media most likely to reach the group
4. factual information appropriate to the group
5. skills for risk reduction
6. motivators for risk reduction
7. intended outcomes (pp. 65–66).

Conclusions Regarding Models, Culture, and Communication

In most of the models examined here, culture is quite implicit. It is interesting that in the numerous studies reviewed by Becker and Joseph (1988), many authors do not report demographic variables, such as race and age. This lack of attention is also noted by Lyons et al. (1990) in their review of AIDS articles in three medical journals. We know, of course, that "demographic variables" do make a difference, as evidenced by the unique findings for particular groups cited here and throughout the literature (also see Flaskerud & Rush, 1989; Nader, Wexler, Patterson, McKusick, & Coates, 1989).

Lip service is given by many working in this area to the importance of culture, but exactly how culture influences the AIDS-related attitudes and practices is not well explicated. Communication is also left unexplicated, although it is clearly central to the preventive process of attitudinal and behavioral change.

A number of studies were found that focus on specific populations, for example drug users (Leukefeld, Battjes, & Amsel, 1990), Black and Hispanic men (Elder-Tabrizy, Wolitski, Rhodes, & Baker, 1991; Peterson & Marin, 1988), and adolescents (DiClemente, Boyer, & Morales, 1988). However, they do not link the descriptions of the groups to specific theoretical frameworks that might guide the development of an effective intervention for a particular group. Others do establish links to theory. For example, Koopman et al. (1990) borrowed from the HBM as well as the concepts of self-efficacy, self-control and peer support. Kelly et al. (1991) described the design and evaluation of a program in the homosexual male community in which key opinion leaders are trained to conduct communicative interventions in the community. Kelly et al. stated that they are working from the diffusion of innovations theory in attempts to develop new community norms, but do not directly cite either the HBM or TRA.

Ross and Rosser (1989) find that education about AIDS fits conceptually with the health behavior models, but in limiting themselves to a monolithic view of gay men, they pay no attention to other notions of culture. The studies they review tell us the obvious, that knowledge is not sufficient for behavior change.

Still others working in this area call for more theoretically driven work. Many of the studies of college student beliefs, attitudes, and practices are not explicitly out of theoretical frameworks, although McDougall and Nelson (1988) work out of the TRA and Leventhal's health behaviors model (Leventhal, Zimmerman, & Gutmann, 1984). Manning et al. (1989) used items straight out of the HBM. Conner et al. (1990) also used the HBM as well as pieces from other theories. Kaemingk and Bootzin (1990) called for the importance of theoretical models but paid no attention to how cultural differences might impact the models or force changes in the conceptual underpinnings. Rugg, O'Reilly, and Galavotti (1990) also mentioned theoretical frames and suggested the importance of the "hard-to-reach" audiences, but again, the argument is not developed.

Scholars working in the area of AIDS prevention seem to be at a crossroads. They have realized that AIDS prevention is dependent on complicated factors, such as ethnicity, gender, age, income, and geographical region. None of the models developed to date place appropriate emphasis on both communication and culture. To continue to be useful, especially to incorporate the concept of education as a cultural communication process, the theoretical models must be married with the grounded descriptions of culture to allow them to have greater descriptive and explanatory power.

INTERCULTURAL COMMUNICATION CONSTRUCTS

Although the scholars publishing in the intercultural communication literature have not focused on issues related to AIDS specifically, or attended to settings that are life-threatening or highly stigmatizing, health communication scholars can benefit from examining the potential utility of intercultural research for HIV education. Specifically, constructs should be explored as to how they might affect the HIV education process and the primary interpersonal processes that are most closely linked with sexual transmission of HIV. In this section we first review several interculturally oriented constructs that HIV educators might find useful in adapting curriculum and presentational approaches to culturally different audiences. Second, we preview several intercultural constructs with implications for managing HIV prevention in sexual relationships.

Gudykunst and Ting-Toomey's (1988) volume, *Culture and Interpersonal Communication,* makes a primary contribution to the intercultural communication literature by tying studies to key communication-centered constructs. They demonstrated the utility of intercultural communication to the larger discipline. Of the constructs Gudykunst and Ting-Toomey reported, several hold potential for informing HIV educational practices. Low and high context communication and ingroup/outgroup relations offer interesting applications to HIV prevention.

Hall's (1976) delineation of culture as high context where "most of the information is in the physical context or is internalized in the person, and little is encoded into the message" (p. 79), has some utility for HIV educators who seek credibility with members of cultures other than their own. The value of the construct will depend on the degree to which the cultural groups have maintained the "cultural attributes" identified with their culture of origin. Thus, if Asian-Americans follow the primary values associated with Eastern cultures, then the high context communication process would telegraph to the educator particular ways to communicate risk information. If, as Hall suggested, the responsibility for understanding or comprehending rests with the interlocutor in the higher context cultures, then HIV prevention messages would be framed differently than they currently are. The U.S. cultural context is described as low, and the primary tendency of educators is to be clear and direct, relatively free of ambiguity. Hence, if members of HIV education audiences represent other than low context communication processes in their own environments, we might question the overall effectiveness of the low context training. Again, for the existing literature on high and low culture to be useful, the degree of assimilation of African-Americans, Latinos, and Asians themselves would require documentation.

Gudykunst and Ting-Toomey (1988) also suggested that the notions of high and low context cultures correlate positively with the dimensions of individualism and collectivism. If we follow this thinking, then, in low context cultures where individualism is dominant, the messages to change health behaviors should include appeals that are salient at the individual level. In high context cultures, the educational program would more appropriately address collective institutions that exert primary influence over the individual. To the extent that Latino culture functions as a modified, collectivistic culture in the United States, there may be interesting parallels to explore.

In examining the "America Responds to AIDS" campaign from the CDC, we do see appeals targeted more pervasively to mothers and the collective institutions, like the church and the family with which traditional Latinas identify. Given the proviso in this chapter against applying monolithic interpretations of culture, we must also caution educators to examine the sociocultural considerations that can trigger individuals to turn away from cultural institutions like the church. For those who are not tied to the institution of the church, it would be important to know if there is great hostility directed toward it, or if the institution is no longer appropriate for them. The "America Responds to AIDS" campaign avoids the church as a controversial institution in that it focuses more on the kindly, concerned grandmother than on the church. Pictorials in the campaign use the church in the background with graphics of a grandmotherly figure wearing a crucifix. Although people may become alienated from the church, the institutions are still a recognized part of the cultural context.

Ingroup and outgroup relationships have been studied extensively in the literature (see Allport, 1954; Bobad & Wallbott, 1986; Cook, 1978; Doise & Sinclair, 1973; Pettigrew, 1986; Williams, 1947). Several issues inherent in the ingroup–outgroup research may have import for studying HIV education. Some cultural groups sustain themselves by assigning positive traits and rewards to their group (ingroup), while assigning unfavorable traits and potential punishments to outside groups. Intergroup contact in itself does not reduce prejudice. Cook (1978), for instance, identified conditions that enable contact to reduce negative stereotyping. Some ingroup–outgroup research identifies fearful reactions to unfamiliar others (Bobad & Wallbott, 1986). In determining whether or not it is advisable to conduct HIV education in a multicultural setting, it may be important to ascertain whether sufficient ingroup bias exists that will disrupt the educational enterprise.

For instance, in urban abuse shelters in Philadelphia the majority of women served are African-Americans. Latinas often leave the shelter because the rules of the shelter function to support the dominant shelter culture (ingroup). If the shelter were able to make gestures to Latinas (outgroup), acknowledging their culturally different parenting practices, some of the ingroup bias might be minimized. Currently, children sleep in separate rooms from their mothers and are required to go to bed much earlier. By altering rules to allow Latinas to have their children with them until they go to sleep, Latinas might be more comfortable and better able to receive HIV education and use shelter services. Examination of ingroup–outgroup relations might bring into sharper focus ways to enhance cultural acceptance among members of different groups, particularly in sites like drug rehabilitation programs and homeless shelters.

Central to understanding how to encourage relational partners to practice risk prevention is the recognition that these partners may have culturally driven verbal and nonverbal relational prescriptions about the amount of talk, the type of talk that is acceptable, and the functions of talk. Several constructs that impinge on the nature of verbal interaction are the elaborate/succinct styles and uncertainty reduction processes of different cultures. HIV education necessarily is responsible for knowing how people negotiate safer sex within the different linguistic parameters that govern talk.

Whether a person's cultural style is to be elaborate, exacting, or succinct affects the degree to which individuals are "able" to offer substantial risk-assessment information. According to Gudykunst and Ting-Toomey (1988), elaborate style is noted for its "rich, expressive language" (p. 105). Exacting style is a conservative estimate of the bare essentials necessary to convey a thought, whereas succinct style incorporates silence, pauses, and understatements. There is considerable evidence that cultures differ on these dimensions. Specific instances cited report differences in intensity of statements, for example, exaggeration between Arabs and Americans (Almaney & Alwan, 1982). Asian cultures often use succinct styles, including silence as a communicative strategy (Johnson & Johnson, 1975). Gudykunst and Ting-Toomey (1988) extrapolate that use of these styles can be correlated with high and low cultural contexts and uncertainty avoidance levels. They suggest that cultures high in uncertainty avoidance and high in context will use more succinct styles, whereas those low in uncertainty avoidance and low in context will use the exacting style, and those with moderate uncertainty avoidance and high context will be elaborators. The viability of these constructs for HIV education will depend on additional work applied to health prevention situations for those at highest risk. Thus, extending these studies to Black and Latino communities and relating them to specific topics, such as sexual negotiation approaches, may yield helpful information for understanding the cultural communication process.

The ability to predict one's own and others' beliefs, attitudes, and behavior in specific settings is tied to the construct of uncertainty reduction (Berger & Calabrese, 1975). The operating assumption is that when uncertainty is reduced understanding can occur. Most of the work in this area has been done in initial interactions, which is appropriate for HIV prevention. Gudykunst and his colleagues (Gudykunst, 1983; Gudykunst, Nishida, & Schmidt, 1988) studied high context cultures and caution in initial interactions and masculine and femininity and uncertainty reduction in same and opposite sex relationships. Although their cross-cultural work is not conclusive, the import of uncertainty reduction as a goal for people of differing cultures interacting in sexual and romantic relationships is worth pursuing. It would be particularly useful to apply this model to at-risk adolescents in urban centers. Adolescents often make choices about actions based on irrational reasoning. If we can assess the tendencies of adolescents to predict the behaviors of their peers within a cultural group, training strategies could incorporate them to reveal the deficits in risky decision making.

TOOLS FOR GATHERING CULTURAL INFORMATION

We have argued throughout this chapter that effective HIV education campaigns and interventions are culturally sensitive, requiring educators and researchers to "know" as much as possible about their intended audiences. Identifying tools for obtaining cultural information about particular groups of people is extremely important. We have also noted the barriers in achieving this knowledge from the intercultural literature and the health behavior change literature specific to HIV. Detailed information-gathering strategies designed to reveal the cultural communication processes of the educator's audience of necessity become part of the research design and operate as formative research tools. As discussed earlier in the models section, some have used brief surveys, ethnographic interviews, discussion groups, and focus groups to gather culture-specific information (Mays & Cochran, 1988; Nyamathi & Shin, 1990). Researchers and educators may also access materials currently being designed by organizations like the American Red Cross for their own training programs that detail the culturally relevant needs of audiences like Black urban teen-agers.

These efforts allow members of a targeted community to dictate what will be effective in that community. If one does not go into the community to observe cultural communication processes and talk to people (i.e., learn the cultural practices that may be relevant to the health message) it is difficult to ensure success. Often this information has been gathered in a piecemeal fashion as health-care professionals report anecdotal stories that may be filtered through the eyes of the reporter. Attempts to standardize formative research has resulted in significant use of focus groups.

In fact, focus group research has exploded in the health field over the past decade. As a formative tool for grounding educational strategies, the focus group has enabled researchers to improve their abilities to more finely hone strategies for reaching particular markets or audiences (Basch, 1987). Two particular programs designed by Blacks Educating Blacks About Sexual Health Issues (BEBASHI) of Philadelphia, a community-based AIDS education organization, exemplify the processes outlined by the National Cancer Institute (1989) to develop health communication programs. This formative technique is but one of those further explicated in Atkin and Freimuth (1989).

The first BEBASHI program was designed by Sanders, Egbuonu, and Hassan (1988). In this initial investigation, three African-American AIDS educators conducted focus groups of African-American teens to define those commonly held beliefs about sexuality, AIDS, condom use, and relationship issues germane to Philadelphia teens in the Black community. This information was then used to design a series of workshops and to produce pamphlets specifically targeted for teens. The workshops were designed to give teens a safe place to understand their own rich Afrocentric history. Based on focus group results, leaders of workshops had group members discuss how relationships happen, the realistic issues about sex that they have to know, and the problems with prevention. They were grounded in the understanding that no one is able to practice prevention 100% of the time. Further, they were encouraged to discover how hard it is to stand up against peer pressure in their own community.

A second project that clearly identifies the cultural process as central to its mission is a project designing HIV education specifically for abused women of color. The project, funded by the American Foundation for AIDS Research (AmFAR), has been overseen by an African-American health educator/manager who has experienced the personal trauma of abuse in a previous marriage. An advisory council consisting of experts from the domestic abuse community was gathered to review the project at each stage. Discussion studies were created for four focus groups conducted with abused women in shelter or drop-in programs and with shelter staff. At all times, focus groups were run by women of color. Transcripts from the focus groups reflect both the language, the world view, the common rituals, and processes connected with domestic abuse in different segments of the African-American community. Thus, at least two cultural transparencies, of African-American culture and the culture of abuse, were used in identifying the core issues of lived experience for African-American women in abusive relationships. From these focus groups, project staff identified six major issues and situations that were most germane to the experiences of these women of color. These issues/situations formed the backdrop for an African-American scriptwriter who transformed the situations into storylines. The scripts were tested with groups of women from the abuse shelter and validated as honest and true to their experiences. Each of the three scripts focuses on a different set of issues and context that reveal the relationship between abuse and HIV and are deeply embedded in the cultural situation of each character. The scenes depict an abusive relationship in the family setting, in a relationship with a substance abuser, and finally with a non-monogamous abusive partner. The scripts were then filmed with actors from an African-American theater company in Philadelphia. Currently, preliminary testing of the videos as an HIV educational tool indicates that the video expressing the cultural values of abused women of color accentuates identification and promotes understanding of the ways abused women use sex as a negotiating tool for survival. It illustrates the extent to which a culture-specific HIV education process can insure cultural integrity in the education process.

CULTURAL DIMENSIONS IN FUTURE RESEARCH

Given our central argument that AIDS education be seen as a cultural communication process, it is appropriate to suggest directions for acknowledging cultural grounding in future research. We hope to identify the lines of research and the methodological shifts necessary to incorporate a cultural perspective. From our perspective as communication researchers, we have selected topics that we feel communication researchers could best address. Our intention here is to identify options for research, not to prioritize their relative importance.

Numerous avenues are available for further exploration of the ways in which culture is embedded in the HIV educational process. Even when using a traditional model of communication such as that used by McGuire (1984), interesting questions emerge when culture is added as an important concept for research. Culture can be included in considerations of destination, source, message, channel, and receiver variables in the creation of health promotion messages.

Destination variables include whether a message is designed to impact knowledge, attitudes, or action; whether a message is to be processed immediately or in the future, and whether it is designed to cause change or cause resistance to change. Although the same factual information can be found in various forms, the two basic AIDS prevention messages are: avoid sharing needles, and do not have unprotected sex. The target audience must be well understood to know which messages will be appropriate in which settings.

AIDS prevention messages and programs typically focus on skills and/or attitudes. Both foci can be enriched by attention to culture. In earlier work, we (Michal-Johnson & Bowen, 1990) noted that a primary tactic for improving HIV education for adolescents in communities of color involves teaching specific communication skills that will increase response efficacy and self-efficacy. They include decision making, peer pressure resistance training, self-inoculation against other messages, changing attitudes (Brooks-Gunn et al., 1988; Flora & Thoresen, 1988), recognizing high-risk behaviors (Haffner, 1988; Shayne & Kaplan, 1988), and interpersonal negotiation skills (Bowen & Michal-Johnson, 1990, 1991; Cvetkovich & Grote, 1981; Oskamp & Mindick, 1983; Shayne & Kaplan,

1988). In other words, recipients must learn verbal and nonverbal communication skills to effectively deal with AIDS-related behaviors. Although communication skills are often presumed to be generalizable across different groups, one research avenue to pursue is whether some skills are more crucial or more appropriate for different cultural groups. For instance, Mays (1989) and Cochran (1989) claimed that the interpersonal negotiation framework may not be realistic for some women of color. Research might also investigate what "counts as" the necessary social support, strategies to regulate one's behavior, and motivations to continue new behaviors (Bandura, 1990) for people in various cultural contexts.

Health promotion advocates realize that knowledge and skills alone will not change behavior; corresponding attitudinal changes must also occur. Attitudes toward behaviors that may be pleasurable but involve high levels of risk must be altered, as must perceived norms among important referent groups (Fishbein & Middlestadt, 1989), and fear resulting from myths and misperceptions about HIV and AIDS. Correcting misinformation is particularly important for the broadly conceived "general public," those perceived to be at low risk for the disease, because of the ways that people will be called on to work with and interact with people who may be HIV positive (Rugg et al., 1990). AIDS intensifies the level of fear and avoidance around topics that are taboo for American culture as a whole (death, sexuality, and homophobia). These taboos also exist for other cultures (see Aoki, Ngin, Mo, & Ja, 1989). Here, then, cultural variation is acknowledged by those who discuss attitude change.

Source variables, involving communicator credibility, attractiveness, power, and the number of communicators used in a message, may also be configured with a cultural transparency. Here again, one must be familiar with the target group to know who will be seen as having credibility. Teachers or doctors may not be as credible as a well-known sports figure to an urban African-American adolescent (but see Kaiser, Manning, & Balson, 1989).

McGuire's schema also includes message variables, such as message style, type of appeal, type of argument, inclusions and omissions of content, organization of message, and use of repetition. Obviously, these are also culturally based because different audiences may respond to a given message in different ways. One example of this is the acceptability of personal testimony as a more credible and persuasive piece of evidence for many African-Americans than for many Whites in this country. Another example to demonstrate how cultural understanding can influence message construction is taken from BEBASHI. BEBASHI outreach educators deliberately promote the use of condoms the next time intercourse takes place. They are aware that attempts to get 100% compliance on condom use for every incident of intercourse are doomed to fail. One can think of numerous experimental designs to test the effectiveness of alternative messages based on group affiliation. If researchers know that a particular strategy is likely to work with a certain group, however, they may face the ethical dilemma of whether to experiment with other messages. Researchers and practitioners alike should be encouraged to continue refining strategies to meet the needs of target groups.

Fourth in this classification are channel variables, which for McGuire include the type of channel (direct vs. mediated, verbal vs. nonverbal), as well as the context for message presentation. Freimuth (1990) and Mays (1989) have recently commented on differential use of media by African-Americans and Latinos. Freimuth noted that radio is underutilized as a channel for dissemination, especially for young audiences, and Mays discussed how choice of channel is related to issues of credibility.

Finally, McGuire pointed out the importance of receiver variables, including the amount of participation desired by audience members, demographic and personality variations, as well as abilities of individuals to follow through on actions. This last group of concerns encompasses many of the variables that the conceptual models discussed earlier attempt to measure, such as normative beliefs and self-efficacy, as well as perceived susceptibility and barriers to action. Freimuth's (1990) study of cancer information details Black cultural beliefs related to health, including conceptualization of time, fatalism, and distrust of dominant institutions. These beliefs provide the backdrop for understanding specific attitudes and beliefs related to AIDS that are relevant when constructing an AIDS education or prevention program targeted to the African-American community. Receiver variables may be particularly important for community level intervention (Coates, 1990). Although receiver variables for some authors, like Freimuth, incorporate attention to cultural variables, in our view, as we have discussed, culture is embedded in all five classes of variables.

CONCLUSION

Equally important to the studies that might arise from attention to the variables addressed by McGuire are the methodological considerations that emerge from this analysis of AIDS education and prevention as a cultural communication process.

First, the theoretical models used for AIDS education need to incorporate culture and communication more explicitly. Work must be done to define which components of the models are culturally influenced. The cultural connection must be more visible in conceptual discussions and the reports of studies that emanate from the models. Many of the extant studies do not include discussions of formative research that might have informed decisions made in developing strategies for use with various targeted populations. It is not clear whether supplementary descriptive research was done, or even if such research was perceived as necessary. Although such formative research may not be particularly expedient, it is nonetheless valuable. What we suggest is in contrast to articles that fail even to report the race, ethnicity, or gender of research participants. In short, we call for a sharper focus on culture to increase the utility and power of the conceptual models.

Second, such changes require an altered mindset, particularly on the part of researchers. We no longer have the luxury of designing studies that fail to account for the cultural diversity that characterizes today's society. Communication researchers have often been criticized for conducting most of their studies on college students, who are not representative of the wider citizenry. Given the trends demonstrated by the Workforce 2000 programs and the attention to cultural diversity even on college campuses, researchers can no longer assume that culture is not important. As we have argued, culture is a system of meanings and practices that affect individuals' attitudes and behaviors. We suggest, then, a metatheoretical shift from the simple pursuit of variables to a more encompassing process of research.

Doing AIDS research is crisis-driven. All those involved in this endeavor are reacting with a sense of urgency to an immediate need. With the taboo issues that often surround perceptions of AIDS, the emotional and moral stakes may be higher. This makes the research different than other health-related issues. Because of these concerns, conscious attention to the cultural aspects of communication is, in our view, of greater value than ignoring culture as peripheral, or worse, irrelevant. Culture is a part of all levels of communication—from the psychological processing of information to the impact of public health campaigns on entire communities.

We offer this caveat to those who would research the communicative dimensions of HIV education: Failure to incorporate culture as a basic underlying epistemological principle can only yield short-sighted findings. Although we acknowledge that explicating relevant cultural factors, issues, and experiences is a time-consuming task, we believe that presuming that culture cannot be adequately clarified through formative research will, in the final analysis, distort well-intentioned campaigns and reduce their overall effectiveness. Finally, overlooking the cultural communication dynamics for a particular group may yield erroneous findings and compromise the academic integrity of the research.

REFERENCES

Aoki, B., Ngin, C. P., Mo, B., & Ja, D. Y. (1989). AIDS prevention models in Asian-American communities. In V. Mays, G. W. Albee, & S. F. Schneider (Eds.), *Primary prevention of AIDS: Psychological approaches* (pp. 290–308). Newbury Park, CA: Sage.

Allport, G. (1954). *The nature of prejudice.* Reading, MA: Addison-Wesley.

Almaney, A., & Alwan, A. (1982). *Communicating with the Arabs.* Prospect Heights, IL: Waveland Press.

Ajzen, I., & Fishbein, M. (1980). *Understanding attitudes and predicting social behavior.* Englewood Cliffs, NJ: Prentice-Hall.

American Red Cross. (1990, October). *African-American HIV/AIDS instructor's manual.* Washington, DC: Author.

Atkin, C., & Freimuth, V. (1989). Formative evaluation research in campaign design. In R. Rice & C. Atkin (Eds.), *Public communication campaigns* (2nd ed., pp. 131–150). Beverly Hills, CA: Sage.

Bandura, A. (1990). Perceived self-efficacy in the exercise of control over AIDS infection. *Evaluation and Program Planning, 13,* 9–17.

Basch, C. E. (1987). Focus group interviews: An underutilized technique for improving theory and practice in health education. *Health Education Quarterly, 14,* 411–448.

Becker, M. H. (Ed.). (1974). *The health belief model and personal health behavior.* Thorofare, NJ: Charles B. Slack.

Becker, M. H., & Joseph, J. G. (1988). AIDS and behavioral change to reduce risk: A review. *American Journal of Public Health, 78,* 394–410.

Berger, C., & Calabrese, R. (1975). Some explorations in initial interactions and beyond: Toward a developmental theory. *Human Communication Research, 1,* 99–112.

Bobad, E., & Wallbott, H. (1986). The effects of social factors on emotional reactions. In K. Sherer, H. Wallbott, & A. Summerfield (Eds.), *Experiencing emotions: A cross-cultural study* (pp. 154–172). Cambridge: Cambridge University Press.

Bowen, S. P., & Michal-Johnson, P. (1990). A rhetorical perspective for HIV education with black urban adolescents. *Communication Research, 17,* 848–866.

Bowen, S. P., & Michal-Johnson, P. (1991). *Evaluating the validity of college students' strategies for HIV risk assessment with relational partners.* Manuscript submitted for publication.

Bowles, J., & Robinson, W. (1989). PHS grants for minority HIV infectious education and prevention efforts. *Public Health Reports, 104,* 552–559.

Brooks-Gunn, J., Boyer, C. B., & Hein, K. (1988). Preventing HIV infection and AIDS in children and adolescents. *American Psychologist, 43,* 958–964.

Catania, J. A., Coates, T. J., Kegeles, S. M., Ekstrand, M., Guydish, J. R., & Bye, L. L. (1989). Implications of the AIDS risk-reduction model for the gay community: The importance of perceived sexual enjoyment and help-seeking behaviors. In V. Mays, G. W. Albee, & S. F. Schneider (Eds.), *Primary prevention of AIDS: Psychological approaches* (pp. 242–261). Newbury Park, CA: Sage.

Catania, J. A., Gibson, D. R., Marin, B., Coates, T. J., & Greenblatt, R. M. (1990). Response bias to assessing sexual behaviors relevant to HIV transmission. *Evaluation and Program Planning, 13,* 19–29.

Centers for Disease Control. (1988, January 29). Guidelines for effective school health education to prevent the spread of AIDS. *Morbidity and Mortality Weekly Report, 37*(No.S-2).

Chu, S., Buehler, J., & Berkelman, L. (1990). Impact of the human immunodeficiency virus epidemic on mortality in women of reproductive age, United States. *Journal of the American Medical Association, 264,* 225–229.

Coates, T. J. (1990). Strategies for modifying sexual behavior for primary and secondary prevention of HIV disease. *Journal of Consulting and Clinical Psychology, 58,* 57–69.

Cochran, S. D. (1989). Women and HIV infection: Issues in prevention and behavior change. In V. Mays, G. W. Albee, & S. F. Schneider (Eds.), *Primary prevention of AIDS: Psychological approaches* (pp. 309–327). Newbury Park, CA: Sage.

Conner, R. F., Mishra, S. I., Lewis, M. A., Bryer, S., Marks, J., Lai, M., & Clark, L. (1990). Theory-based evaluation of AIDS-related knowledge, attitudes, and behavior changes. *New Directions for Program Evaluation, 46,* 75–84.

Cook, S. (1978). Interpersonal and attitudinal outcomes in cooperating interracial groups. *Journal of Research and Development in Education, 12,* 97–113.

Cvetkovich, G., & Grote, B. (1981). Psychosocial maturity and teenage contraceptive use: An investigation of decision-making and communication skills. *Population & Environment, 4,* 211–226.

Dalton, H. L. (1989). AIDS in blackface. *Daedelus, 118,* 205–227.

De La Cancela, V. (1989). Minority AIDS prevention: Moving beyond cultural perspectives towards sociopolitical empowerment. *AIDS Education and Prevention, 1,* 141–153.

DiClemente, R. J., Boyer, C. B., & Morales, E. S. (1988). Minorities and AIDS: Knowledge, attitudes, and misconceptions among black and Latino adolescents. *American Journal of Public Health, 78,* 55–77.

Doise, W., & Sinclair, A. (1973). The categorization of process in intergroup relations. *European Journal of Social Psychology, 3,* 145–157.

Elder-Tabrizy, K. A., Wolitski, R. J., Rhodes, F., & Baker, J. G. (1991). AIDS and competing health concerns of blacks, Hispanics, & whites. *Journal of Community Health, 16*(1), 11–21.

Fishbein, M., & Middlestadt, S. E. (1989). Using the theory of reasoned action as a framework for understanding and changing AIDS-related behaviors. In V. Mays, G. W. Albee, & S. F. Schneider (Eds.), *Primary prevention of AIDS: Psychological approaches* (pp. 93–110). Newbury Park, CA: Sage.

Flaskerud, J. H., & Nyamathi, A. M. (1989). Black and Latina women's AIDS related knowledge, attitudes, and practices. *Research in Nursing and Health, 12,* 339–346.

Flaskerud, J. H., & Rush, C. E. (1989). AIDS and traditional health beliefs and practices of black women. *Nursing Research, 38,* 210–215.

Flora, J. A., & Thoresen, C. E. (1988). Reducing the risk of AIDS in adolescents. *American Psychologist, 43,* 965–970.

Freimuth, V. S. (1990). *Narrowing the cancer knowledge gap among blacks.* Report prepared for the National Cancer Institute, Bethesda, MD.

Geertz, C. (1973). *The interpretation of cultures.* New York: Basic Books.

Gudykunst, W. (1983). *Intercultural communication theory.* Beverly Hills, CA: Sage.

Gudykunst, W., Nishida, T., & Schmidt, K. (1988, May). *Cultural personality and relational influences on uncertainty reduction in ingroup vs. outgroup and same- vs. opposite-sex relationships.* Paper presented at the International Communication Association, New Orleans.

Gudykunst, W., & Ting-Toomey, S. (1988). *Culture and interpersonal communication.* Beverly Hills, CA: Sage.

Haffner, D. W. (1988). AIDS and adolescents: School health education must begin now. *Journal of School Health, 58,* 154–155.

Hall, E. (1976). *Beyond culture.* New York: Doubleday.

Janz, N., & Becker, M. (1984). The health belief model: A decade later. *Health Education Quarterly, 11,* 1–47.

Johnson, C., & Johnson, F. (1975). Interaction rules and ethnicity. *Social Forces, 54,* 452–466.

Kaemingk, K. L., & Bootzin, R. R. (1990). Behavior change strategies for increasing condom use. *Evaluation and Program Planning, 13,* 47–54.

Kaiser, M. A., Manning, D. T., & Balson, P. M. (1989). Lay volunteers' knowledge and beliefs about AIDS prevention. *Journal of Community Health, 14,* 215–226.

Kelly, J. A., St. Lawrence, J. S., Diaz, Y. E., Stevenson, L. Y., Hauth, A. C., Basfield, T. L., Kalichman, S. C., Smith, J. E., & Andrew, M. E. (1991). HIV risk behavior reduction following intervention with key opinion leaders of population: An experimental analysis. *American Journal of Public Health, 81,* 168–171.

Kirscht, J. P., & Joseph, J. G. (1989). The health belief model: Some implications for behavior change with reference to homosexual males. In V. Mays, G. W. Albee, & S. F. Schneider (Eds.), *Primary prevention of AIDS: Psychological approaches* (pp. 111–127). Newbury Park, CA: Sage.

Koopman, C., Rotheram-Borus, M. J., Henderson, R., Bradley, J. S., & Hunter, J. (1990). Assessment of knowledge of AIDS and beliefs about AIDS prevention among adolescents. *AIDS Education and Prevention, 2,* 58–69.

Leukefeld, C. G., Battjes, R. J., & Amsel, Z. (Eds.). (1990). *AIDS and intravenous drug use: Future directions for community-based prevention research.* (Research Monograph No. 93; DHHS Publication No. ADM 90-1627.) Washington, DC: National Institute on Drug Abuse.

Leventhal, H., Zimmerman, R., & Gutmann, M. (1984). Compliance: A self-regulation perspective. In D. Gentry (Ed.), *Handbook of behavioral medicine* (pp. 369–436). New York: Guilford.

Longshore, D. (1990). AIDS education for three high risk populations. *Evaluation and Program Planning, 13,* 67–72.

Lyons, J. S., Larson, D. B., Bareta, J. C., Lu, I., Anderson, A., & Sparks, C. (1990). A systematic analysis of the quantity of AIDS publications and the quality of research methods in three general medical journals. *Evaluation and Program Planning, 13,* 73–77.

Maibach, E. (1989, May). *Using social cognitive theory for the development of AIDS prevention videos.* Paper presented at the annual meeting of the Speech Communication Association, San Francisco.

Manning, D. T., Barenberg, N., Gallese, L., & Rice, J. C. (1989). College students' knowledge and health beliefs about AIDS: Implications for AIDS education and prevention. *Journal of American College Health, 37,* 254–259.

Mays, V. M. (1989). AIDS prevention in black populations: Methods of a safer kind. In V. Mays, G. W. Albee, & S. F. Schneider (Eds.), *Primary prevention of AIDS: Psychological approaches* (pp. 264–279). Newbury Park, CA: Sage.

Mays, V. M., & Cochran, S. D. (1988). Issues in the perception of AIDS risk and risk reduction activities by black and Hispanic/Latina women. *American Psychologist, 43,* 949–957.

McDougall, K. H., & Nelson, G. S. (1988, May). *Communication, persuasion, and AIDS prevention.* Paper presented to the Annual Conference of the Speech Communication Association, New Orleans.

McGuire, W. J. (1984). Public communication as a strategy for inducing health-promoting behavioral change. *Preventive Medicine, 13,* 299–319.

Michal-Johnson, P. (1988, February). *Clinician's interpretations of STD client's needs.* Paper presented at the International Communication Association Mid-Year Health Conference, Monterey, CA.

Michal-Johnson, P., & Bowen, S. P. (1990). *AIDS discourse in the romantic relationships of college students.* Manuscript submitted for publication.

Montgomery, S. B., Joseph, J. G., Becker, M. H., Ostrow, D. G., Kessler, R. C., & Kirscht, J. P. (1989). The health belief model in understanding compliance with preventive recommendations for AIDS: How useful? *AIDS Education and Prevention, 1,* 303–323.

Mumby, D. K. (1989). Ideology and the social construction of meaning: A communication perspective. *Communication Quarterly, 37,* 291–304.

Nader, P. R., Wexler, D. B., Patterson, T. L., McKusick, L., & Coates, T. (1989). Comparison of beliefs about AIDS among urban, suburban, incarcerated and gay adolescents. *Journal of Adolescent Health Care, 10,* 413–418.

National Cancer Institute. (1989). *Making health communication programs work: A planner's guide* (NIH Publication No. 89-1493). Bethesda, MD: Office of Cancer Communications.

Nyamathi, A., & Shin, D. M. (1990). Designing a culturally sensitive educational program for black and Hispanic women of childbearing age. *NAACOG's Clinical Issues in Perinatal and Women's Health Nursing, 1*(1), 86–98.

Nyamathi, A., Shuler, P., & Porche, M. (1990). AIDS educational program for minority women at risk. *Family & Community Health, 13*(2), 54–64.

Oskamp, S., & Mindick, B. (1983). Personality and attitudinal barriers to contraception. In D. Byrne & W. Fisher (Eds.), *Adolescents, sex and contraception* (pp. 66–107). Hillsdale, NJ: Lawrence Erlbaum Associates.

Peterson, J., & Marin, G. (1988). Issues in the prevention of AIDS among Black and Hispanic men. *American Psychologist, 43,* 871–877.

Pettigrew, T. (1986). The intergroup contact hypothesis reconsidered. In M. Hewstone & R. Brown (Eds.), *Contact and conflict in intergroup encounters.* Oxford: Basil Blackwell.

Rosenstock, I. (1974). Historical origins of the health belief model. *Health Education Monographs, 2,* 328–335.

Ross, M. W., & Rosser, B. R. S. (1989). Education and AIDS risks: A review. *Health Education Research: Theory and Practice, 4,* 273–284.

Rugg, D. L., O'Reilly, K. R., & Galavotti, C. (1990). AIDS prevention evaluation: Conceptual and methodological issues. *Evaluation and Program Planning, 13,* 79–89.

Sanders, L., Egbuonu, L., & Hassan, R. (1988, June). *Refining education messages targeted to inner-city youth.* Paper presented at the Fourth International Conference on AIDS, Stockholm.

Schneider, D. (1976). Notes toward a theory of culture. In K. H. Busso & H. A. Selby (Eds.), *Meaning in anthropology* (pp. 197–220). Albuquerque, NM: University of New Mexico Press.

Servaes, J. (1989). Cultural identity and modes of communication. In J. A. Anderson (Ed.), *Communication yearbook 12* (pp. 386–434). Newbury Park, CA: Sage.

Shayne, V. T., & Kaplan, B. J. (1988). AIDS education for adolescents. *Youth and Society, 20,*180–208.

Solomon, M. Z., & DeJong, W. (1986). Recent sexually transmitted disease prevention efforts and their implications for AIDS health education. *Health Education Quarterly, 13,* 301–316.

Turner, V. W. (1974). *Dramas, fields, and metaphors: Symbolic action in human society.* Ithaca, NY: Cornell University Press.

Williams, R. (1947). *Reduction in intergroup tensions.* New York: Social Science Press.

Witte, K. (in press). Preventing AIDS through persuasive communications: A framework for constructing effective preventive health messages. In F. Korzenny & S. Ting-Toomey (Eds.), *International and intercultural annual.* Annandale, VA: Speech Communication Association.

CHAPTER NINE

AIDS and the Media Agenda

James W. Dearing
Michigan State University

Everett M. Rogers
University of Southern California

During the mid-1980s many Americans misunderstood the risks associated with AIDS transmission (Roper Center for Public Opinion Research Archives, 1983–1990; Singer & Rogers, 1987; Singer, Rogers, & Corcoran, 1987). This widespread misunderstanding has been attributed to scientists and authority figures (Scott, 1987), journalists (Brecher, 1988; Shaw, 1987a, 1987b), copyeditors and media decision makers (Dorfman, 1987; Kinsella, 1988, 1989; Kramer, 1988; Shilts, 1987), organizations (Perrow & Guillen, 1990), and the triumvirate institutions of science, government, and journalism (Check, 1987). The problem of disseminating accurate information about AIDS to the public was somewhat indicative of the problems of risk communication about health issues in general (Plough & Krimsky, 1987).

All of these explanations at least partly indict the performance of mass media organizations. Yet none of the proponents of these criticisms suggest the extent to which mass media organizations are bound in certain relations that inhibit their ability to better communicate risk. We do not imply that mass media organizations should be exonerated for their flawed performance in AIDS coverage in the United States. But we do suggest that the symbiotic nature of interdependencies in which news organizations necessarily participate importantly determines their ability to communicate information about risk. This chapter suggests the factors that influenced the importance of AIDS on the mass media news agenda in (a) San Francisco, and (b) the United States, through 1988. We follow a suggestion by Atkin and Arkin (1990) that an important research priority for understanding how the mass media cover public health issues should be the critical study of exogenous and endogenous influences on the determination of what is considered news.

MEDIA AGENDA-SETTING

Scholars have long regarded the mass media news agenda as an important topic of study (Lazarsfeld & Merton, 1948), and calls have been sounded for more research on how the media agenda is set (Chaffee, 1980). Yet media agenda-setting has been relatively neglected by scholars, compared to the study of either public agenda-setting (in which the public agenda is the dependent variable of study) or policy agenda-setting (in which the issue agenda of policymakers is the dependent variable of study; Rogers & Dearing, 1988; Shoemaker & Reese, 1991). We propose that one reason for the lack of study of media agenda-setting is the difficulty of conceptualizing and operationalizing how media agenda-setting can be quantified.

Quantification of the influences on the news agenda of media organizations is confounded partly because of the difficulty in operationalizing certain influences as either endogenous or exogenous. Endogenous influences on news agendas are variables that originate from within a mass media organization, such as the perceptions of a news issue by editors. Exogenous influences on news agendas are variables that originate from outside mass media organizations, such as the number of protest marches held about a topic. Endogenous and exogenous influences are not mutually exclusive. For example, communication scholars have long suggested that media decision makers implicitly and explicitly apply a set of criteria against which potential news issues are judged. These criteria include sensation, conflict, mystery, celebrity, deviance, tragedy, and proximity (Shoemaker, with Mayfield, 1987), the "breaking quality" of a news issue, how new information can be molded to recast old issues in a new way (Rogers, Dearing, & Chang, 1991), and the degree to which new information can be fit into existing constructs (Meyer, 1990). These newsworthiness criteria, when applied by people within news organizations to an issue, become endogenous determinants of news attention. But issues are already laden with meanings prior to receiving news coverage. Presidents, members of Congress, political action committees, and all other types of issue proponents seek to identify their issues with certain news criteria and to control the ways in which their issues are understood and interpreted in the news. Journalists may assign new criteria and meanings to issues (endogenous influence), or they may simply communicate the criteria and meanings already given to issues (exogenous influence). This confounded nature of the influences on media news agendas makes distinctions between variables as endogenous or exogenous somewhat facile, and suggests that qualitative methods may be better suited to understanding media agenda influences.

The study of media agenda-setting is essentially the study of the distribution and use of power and influence in society (Reese, 1991). All issues arise either from the environment or from people, and those issues that arise from the environment are usually rapidly adopted by issue champions. The competition among issues for a place on the news agenda is really a competition among people in obtaining news attention for their issues (Mansbach & Vasquez, 1981). Here, we concentrate on the degree to which different variables had an impact on the amount of news coverage given to the issue of AIDS. For example, a government health official who repeatedly proclaims AIDS to be a runaway epidemic would increase the amount of news coverage given to AIDS.

The present analysis shows that mass media organizations are far from autonomous actors in the determination of what is news. The actions of media organizations and their employees are constricted by networks of institutional, social, and work relationships. For example, Linsky (1986), in a study of the pervasiveness of the mass media in U.S federal policymaking, shows that federal policymakers need mass media news coverage to arouse support for their initiatives, whereas journalists need to maintain good relations with policymakers in order to ensure access to new information about the government. Linsky argued that the media–policy relationship is better characterized by symbiosis, or mutual reliance and need, than competition, adversity, or outright conflict.

The present analysis focuses on interdependent relations among mass media organizations, policymakers, and publics. Interdependency is the symbiotic reliance of two or more social units with each other. Media organizations exist in complementary interdependencies (Ball-Rokeach, 1985; Qualter, 1985), which is why agenda-setting research often shows mutual or indeterminant causality of issue salience among the media, the public, and policymakers, and why meta-reviews of such research suggest contradictions or contingencies (Rogers & Dearing, 1988). Accordingly, this analysis focuses on how news attention to the issue of AIDS was the product of symbiotic relations over which the mass media have only limited control.

THE ISSUE OF AIDS IN SAN FRANCISCO

Although New York City has the largest number of AIDS cases, San Francisco has the most AIDS-infected individuals per million population (Centers for Disease Control, 1988). San Francisco had a population of

749,000 in 1986, making it the 12th largest city in the United States. The city is compact geographically, measuring about 7 by 7 miles. This high population density, along with several forms of mass transit and limited parking spaces for automobiles, contributes to the city being socially close-knit. Important local news travels fast via interpersonal communication channels in San Francisco.

The city is governed by a mayor and 10 supervisors, all currently elected at large. San Francisco's mayor and the 10 supervisors were all Democrats. The mayor has the power to sign or veto fiscal initiatives. Compared with other U.S. cities, San Francisco's population is liberal and progressive, and displays a "live and let live" philosophy, with tolerance for diverse lifestyles.

In 1974, police harassment of gay men was halted by the city government (Fitzgerald, 1986). This "coming of rights" was important for the already large gay and lesbian population of the city. San Francisco became a place where gays could publicly declare their sexual orientation without fear of reprisal. Word spread in gay newspapers across the United States that San Francisco was the place to live. Between 1974 and 1982, approximately 5,000 gays per year moved to the city. New arrivals settled in "the Castro," a one-by-one-half-mile district, making it the center of gay life. A less visible gay concentration developed in affluent Pacific Heights, and Polk Street became the strip for male prostitutes. Gay bathhouses flourished on Folsom Street. The 1982 gay population of San Francisco was estimated at about 100,000 (S. Dritz, personal communication, October 15, 1987); two out of every five men in San Francisco are gay. The gay population was the most formidable voting bloc in San Francisco, although it was split into conservative and liberal factions. Six out of 10 gay and bisexual men held college degrees, and their incomes were higher than San Franciscans in general (San Francisco AIDS Foundation, 1987a).

Initiating the Agenda-Setting Process in San Francisco

Beginning in 1978, the epidemiology of AIDS was foreshadowed by a similar rise in the number of Hepatitis B patients, a disease that does not have the long dormancy period of the AIDS virus. Epidemiologists, however, had no way of knowing that another, more serious disease was being concomitantly spread (S. Dritz, personal communication, October 15, 1987). Between 1982 and 1987, more than 20,000 to 25,000 gays moved out of San Francisco as a result of the AIDS epidemic, while 2,500 died of the disease.

Gay medical doctors acted in a primordial role in responding to the first signs of the epidemic. Gay physicians immediately interpreted the first cases of immune suppression as a public health threat. In early 1981, word spread throughout the San Francisco medical community of the strange immunity problem of otherwise healthy young gay men. What was a mystery to the U.S. population in the early 1980s was frighteningly real to San Franciscans. The effects of the disease were severe, dilapidating the body's natural immune defenses, and laying victims open to attack by a variety of diseases that the human body could normally repel. Working closely with the San Francisco Department of Public Health, gay and nongay physicians made the AIDS issue a priority. "Our grass roots health communication played a huge role," a local epidemiologist said. "Together, through our network with the medical community and gay communities, we were able to make this issue swell locally" (S. Dritz, personal communication, October 15, 1987).

Ideologically, some gays in San Francisco tried to protect their newfound freedom to live "out of the closet" by initially opposing public health initiatives against the disease, such as attempts to close the gay bathhouses. These gays interpreted aggressive attempts to stop the spread of the HIV virus as violations of their individual civil rights.

Nonprofit community-based groups played an important early role in raising consciousness and clearing up confusion about AIDS in San Francisco. These local organizations are largely staffed by volunteers, many of whom are gay. In 1987, a media resource guide on AIDS information listed 87 clinics, support groups, task forces, institutes, and associations that dealt in various ways with AIDS (San Francisco AIDS Foundation, 1987b). During fiscal year 1984–1985, the three largest of these organizations in San Francisco provided more than 80,000 hours of social support and counseling services for AIDS victims, responded to over 30,000 telephone inquiries, and distributed almost 250,000 pieces of AIDS-related literature. These organizations typically began as volunteer groups, and then attracted city, state, or federal funding. The city government of San Francisco provided 62% of the financial support for these groups during their early years (Arno, 1986). A 1987 survey in San Francisco showed that 89% of gay and bisexual male respondents had contributed time and/or money to a San Francisco AIDS-related organization (San Francisco AIDS Foundation, 1987a).

The gay men's groups recruited individuals on the streets of San Francisco and through friendship networks to participate in small educational meetings in which the nature of AIDS was explained and in which methods of safer sex were promoted. A series of annual surveys of gay men in San Francisco showed that the rate of spread of HIV slowed gradually until it was only 1% or 2% by 1989. However, by then, about 70% of all gay men in San Francisco had the HIV virus (San Francisco AIDS Foundation, 1987a).

Setting the Media Agenda in San Francisco

The several gay and lesbian weekly newspapers in San Francisco provided a forum within which conservative and liberal gays attempted to define the issue of AIDS for their community. The editor of the city's largest circulation (30,000) gay newspaper, the *Bay Area Reporter,* felt that AIDS coverage was, after 1981, comprehensive and objective (B. Jones, personal communication, October 15, 1987). Yet bathhouses, where much unsafe, promiscuous sex took place, were important advertisers in the *Reporter,* thus providing an economic incentive against alerting readers to the dangers of AIDS or editorializing in favor of closing the bathhouses (Shilts, 1987). Perhaps because of this influence, Bay Area gay papers tended to argue against closure of the bathhouses.

Although gay newspapers led the general circulation newspapers and television stations in AIDS coverage in San Francisco (H. G. Britt, personal communication, October 15, 1987; B. Jones, personal communication, October 15, 1987), our personal interviews with San Francisco media officials suggest that gatekeepers at the major mass media did not follow the gay press closely. Local gay newspapers did not play an agenda-setting role for the AIDS issue for the major mass media in San Francisco. But the gay newspapers did alert the gay population of San Francisco to the dangerous new epidemic, even if the gay papers were by and large not advocating drastic public health precautions, such as closing the bathhouses.

The *San Francisco Chronicle* is credited with the most comprehensive coverage of the AIDS issue in the United States (Altman, 1986; Shilts, 1987). Our analysis shows that the *San Francisco Chronicle* published more articles about AIDS than did *The New York Times, Los Angeles Times,* or *Washington Post* from 1981 to 1988 (Dearing & Rogers, 1988; Rogers et al., 1991).

Why did the *Chronicle* publish so many articles about AIDS? A former city editor in 1982 decided that his paper should hire a gay reporter, and Randy Shilts, author of a subsequent book about AIDS, was recruited. Although the *San Francisco Chronicle* continued to print articles from the wire services, and important articles written by science editor David Perlman and reporter Charles Petit, Shilts was soon covering AIDS full time. Many of Shilts' articles were not journalistically objective (e.g., he advocated the closing of the bathhouses), and local gays complained about his editorializing within news articles. But Shilts was committed to changing the behavior of the gay community. At that time, in late 1982, Shilts was the nation's only full-time AIDS reporter.

One San Francisco television station devoted considerable airtime to the AIDS issue, relative to other Bay Area television stations. KPIX-TV aired its first AIDS special in 1983. Largely on the initiative of one reporter, Jim Bunn, KPIX broadcast over 1,000 of its own news reports on AIDS over the 4-year period from 1983 to 1987 (KPIX, 1987). KPIX also produced more than 60 public service announcements (PSAs) about AIDS prevention, financed an AIDS hotline in the city, and contributed the cost of publishing information pamphlets on AIDS. The television station's AIDS coverage earned a Presidential Citation, a regional Emmy, a Peabody Award, and a National Emmy for Community Service. The station's AIDS programs were widely syndicated throughout the nation (Hogan, 1988). KPIX-TV's extensive coverage served its own organizational goals as well. The station's parent corporation, Group W Television, required that each of its stations devote a small portion of its programming to community service issues, and KPIX-TV's general manager had been under pressure to find such an issue. AIDS fit the bill. Fortuitously, the enormity of the issue locally and KPIX's early decision to pour resources into covering the AIDS issue paid off in terms of massive local publicity for the station.

Did local newspapers put the issue of AIDS on the television agenda, or vice versa? Oftentimes, television news personnel use morning newspapers as a starting place to decide which news stories to cover. We could find no evidence that local television responded to local newspaper coverage of AIDS in any patterned way, or vice versa. Our interviews at both the *San Francisco Chronicle* and at KPIX-TV suggest that each was largely unaware of the other's AIDS coverage. The considerable coverage given to the AIDS issue by the local and national gay press, local newspapers, and television stations in San Francisco, gradually put the issue of AIDS on the public agenda. Constant media exposure, along with pressure from the gay public in San Francisco, pushed the issue of AIDS onto the desks of policymakers in San Francisco's City Hall.

Former Mayor Diane Feinstein is the daughter of a medical doctor, and was married to a physician. When Feinstein finally understood the ramifications of AIDS, she interpreted the problem as a public health issue worthy of government municipal funding, although she had been attempting to cut health-care costs in the city (H. G. Britt, personal communication, October 15, 1987). The mayor also favored direct action like closing the gay bathhouses, a position that alienated conservative gays. Liberal gays were similarly alienated by Feinstein's veto of gay Supervisor Harry Britt's Domestic Partner's Ordinance. Feinstein, who championed gay rights more than any other top public official in the nation (Shilts, 1987), found herself in a maelstrom of gay politics. "We had to educate Diane about gay lifestyles," said Britt. "Imagine explaining this to a woman who thought gay bathhouses were a place to go take a bath" (H. G. Britt, personal communication, October 15, 1987).

By 1983, Feinstein was heavily involved in the municipal government's battle against the AIDS epidemic. Her signature on a $450,000 appropriation authorized the city to finance the world's first AIDS clinic, grief counseling, and a personal support network for AIDS patients, as well as the first city-funded educational program about AIDS in the United States. At that time, nearly 20% of all the funding in the United States for fighting AIDS was authorized in San Francisco (Shilts, 1987). The city, through its Department of Public Health and two major hospitals, along with services contracted to the Shanti Project (for patient care) and to the Kaposi's Sarcoma Foundation (later the San Francisco AIDS Foundation) for education, was universally hailed as the most progressive municipal government for AIDS education and treatment. Supervisor Britt did not feel that he was responding to media pressure when he sponsored funding proposals for AIDS treatment and education. "We have constituents dying," Britt said. "They talk to us. I think I responded to the public and to the disease itself" (H. G. Britt, personal communication, October 15, 1987). A source within the San Francisco Department of Public Health felt that the department pushed the city's Board of Supervisors, as well as the mayor. The mayor, she added, was politically very aware of her gay constituents (S. Dritz, personal communication, October 15, 1987). Public officials in San Francisco were responding to a serious health crisis in their largest, most politically sophisticated constituency. No city politician could ignore the gay voters of San Francisco. Indeed, there was no dissension about AIDS spending proposals at San Francisco city council meetings. If the AIDS epidemic had been concentrated in an identifiable demographic category in San Francisco other than gays, policy responses to AIDS probably would likely not have been as prompt. This situation was just the opposite of what was occurring at the national level.

THE SLOW-ONSET NATURE OF THE AIDS ISSUE IN THE UNITED STATES

A rapidly spreading disease that has an extremely high mortality rate might be expected to have attracted swift attention by the national mass media, the public, and by U.S. policymakers. However, the issue of AIDS did not diffuse nearly as rapidly as the disease itself. Whereas organized responses in San Francisco by medical personnel, interest groups, the local media, and politicians met the challenge of AIDS early, organized responses did not characterize how the United States as a whole responded to the disease.

Each year in the United States a few potential issues become public;

the vast majority die an unheralded death by failing to attract sufficient mass media attention. If a scientific issue is not in the mass media, then it is not news, and if it is not news, then it does not become a public issue. AIDS did not make it onto the U.S. mass media news agenda for 4 years. For example, during 1981 and 1982, very little mass media attention was given to the AIDS epidemic, although the Centers for Disease Control (CDC) reported over 800 AIDS cases diagnosed and over 350 deaths by the end of 1982. After a brief flurry of news stories about AIDS in mid-1983, media interest in the topic subsided, and relatively few news stories appeared for the next 22 months, until July 1985. For the first 48 months of the AIDS epidemic, a point at which 9,944 individuals had AIDS (according to CDC statistics), the issue of AIDS was still not on the media agenda.

The mass media, especially television, are adept at covering quick-onset issues, such as earthquakes, but less inclined to give news attention to slow-onset issues (such as AIDS) or trends (such as the number of deaths from AIDS). Mass media decision makers have difficulty with, or are reluctant in packaging, a slow-onset issue into "news bites." The mass media appetite is primed for quick-onset issues that can be reported, categorized, understood, and forgotten just as the next news issue arises. AIDS did not fit this pattern. The disease was difficult to report, it defied easy categorization, it was little understood (even by scientists), and it would not go away.

Scientific publications played a direct but short-lived agenda-setting role for early major mass media coverage of the AIDS issue. For example, the first article in the four major newspapers we analyzed (the *Washington Post, Los Angeles Times, The New York Times,* and *San Francisco Chronicle*) on what was later called "AIDS" was carried on June 5, 1981, in the *Los Angeles Times,* on page A3. It resulted directly from the CDC issue of *Morbidity & Mortality Weekly Report,* dated June 5. The *San Francisco Chronicle* published its first article one day later. The first article in *The New York Times* appeared almost 1 month later, on July 3, page A20 (it also resulted directly from a CDC report). The next articles about AIDS in each newspaper appeared in early July, again based directly on a CDC report. Later in 1981, scientific articles about AIDS in the December 10 issue of the *New England Journal of Medicine* led directly to an article in each of our four newspapers of study. Throughout the 1980s, medical and science journals continued as an important source for mass media news reports about AIDS. From June 1981 through February 1988, the *Journal of the American Medical Association* published 639 articles about AIDS, the *New England Journal of Medicine* published 378 articles about AIDS, *Science* published 169 articles about AIDS, and *Mortality & Morbidity Weekly Report* published 128 articles about AIDS. So a huge scientific literature on AIDS was rapidly beginning to accumulate.

Mass Media Coverage of AIDS in the U.S.

We analyzed both (a) the distribution of all news stories about AIDS over time, and (b) the themes of these stories, printed in the *Washington Post,* the *Los Angeles Times, The New York Times,* and the *San Francisco Chronicle,* and broadcast on the network nightly news programs of ABC, NBC, and CBS, from mid-1981 through 1988.

Both the distribution of news stories and the themes of the stories were highly and positively correlated among these seven media of study (Dearing & Rogers, 1988; Rogers et al., 1991). Nevertheless, important differences in their portrayal of the disease existed among at least two of these news organizations. For example, the *San Francisco Chronicle* (a) ran more stories about AIDS, (b) earlier, and (c) from a more humanistic slant, by focusing on victims, than did the other six media organizations we studied. *The New York Times'* coverage of AIDS was (a) late and (b) incomplete, for the first 4 years of the epidemic, but then (c) rapidly caught up and surpassed most other mass media in both the quantity and quality of its reporting on AIDS. Indeed, the general picture of late and flawed media coverage of AIDS would be incomplete without mentioning the few counter-examples of virtuous, heroic, dogged journalists, such as Laurie Garrett of National Public Radio (Kinsella, 1989; Klaidman & Beauchamp, 1987).

The content of the stories about AIDS can, in general, be divided into (a) an initial era of the "mysterious new gay plague" (June 1981 through April 1983); (b) a science era, during which medical sources and hypotheses about disease transmission dominated news stories (May 1983 through June 1985); (c) a human era, during which AIDS became an issue of common concern through the disease's personification and perceived relevance to general audiences (July 1985 through January 1987); and (d) a political era, during which stories were dominated by public policy controversy (February 1987 through December 1988).

Mid-1985 was the turning point at which mass media editors interpreted AIDS to be a very important issue (see Fig. 9.1). The death of movie actor Rock Hudson and, especially, the public prejudice against schoolboy Ryan White in Kokomo, Indiana, caught the interest of mass media decision makers, who ran numerous news stories centered around these tragedies. Prior to Rock Hudson's death in October 1985, U.S. policymakers and the public could have concluded from mass media coverage that AIDS was perversely fascinating, but, overall, not very important as a national issue. The Hudson and White events helped humanize the AIDS issue,

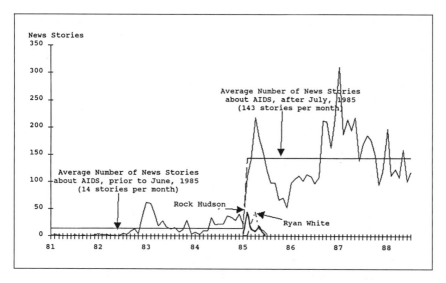

FIG. 9.1. The impact of the Rock Hudson and Ryan White news events on the number of news stories about the issue of AIDS (from June 1981 through December 1988).

and thus changed the meaning of the epidemic for media news people (Rogers et al., 1991). These two stories popularized the issue of AIDS and led editors to interpret AIDS as an issue that was of interest and relevance to general audiences (Check, 1987).

Role of *The New York Times*

The impact of *The New York Times* on the importance of AIDS on the national mass media agenda is not so much a function of the *Times'* news article content per se, but rather the salience and credibility that other media decision makers attribute to the issues that *The New York Times* chooses to cover. For international and often for domestic news, *The New York Times* sets the news agenda of other U.S. mass media. For example, when Jerry Bishop, medical writer for the *Wall Street Journal* since 1958, proposed that the *Journal* should cover the story, he figured that his own reluctant editors wondered, "If it's [AIDS] such a big thing, why isn't *The New York Times* covering it?" (quoted by Shaw, 1987a).

Initially, *The New York Times* paid little attention to AIDS. The newspaper published its first page 1 story about AIDS on May 25, 1983. This date was 12 months later than the *Los Angeles Times,* 10 months later than the *Washington Post,* 11 months after the *Philadelphia Inquirer,* and 11 months after the *San Francisco Chronicle* (Shaw, 1987a).

The newspaper's management did not consider AIDS to be newsworthy from 1981 to mid-1985. When Max Frankel became executive editor in late 1985, coverage of AIDS expanded dramatically.

The amount of attention given to AIDS by the four major newspapers that we studied were the result of organizational and personal variables. A former editor at *The New York Times* remained long unconvinced that stories on gays were appropriate for his newspaper. For several years into the AIDS epidemic, the *Times* refused to use the word "gay" except within quoted passages. Reporters would shelve news leads on gay issues because articles on gay issues had little chance to appear on page A1 (B. Nelson, personal communication, October 15, 1987). The reward system for star reporters hinges directly on their number of front-page articles; articles appearing elsewhere in the newspaper do not count for so much (Winsten, 1985).

Lawrence Altman, science writer for the *Times* and a former CDC employee, offered other reasons why the *Times* was not in the vanguard on reporting about the disease. Altman was aware, in early 1981, of a disease in New York's gay community, and he was preparing to write a story about it. Then he was distracted by a more important story, the medical aspects of the Reagan assassination attempt. Soon afterward, he was assigned to cover the assassination attempt on Pope John Paul II, in Rome. While overseas, Altman broke both of his elbows, and could not write for a number of weeks. So science reporting of the new gay disease in *The New York Times* was slowed (Altman, 1987). The intense competition at major news organizations often discourages writers from passing story leads to fellow employees (Winsten, 1985).

According to our analysis, from 1981 to 1987, the number of articles about AIDS in *The New York Times* clustered around spectacular events. More articles appeared in the *Times* when sensational, human interest AIDS stories were in the news, relative to our other three major newspapers of study. When sensational news stories were not dominating the AIDS issue, the *Times* published fewer articles on AIDS, relative to the other three newspapers of study. For example, after a May 6, 1983, press release from the *Journal of the American Medical Association* (JAMA) carried comments by a medical scientist at the National Institutes of Health that a new study implicated "routine household contact" as a means of AIDS transmission, the number of AIDS-related articles in *The New York Times* increased from 1 article in April, to 21 in May, 29 in June, 23 in July, and to 12 in August, before settling back to 6 in September 1983 (scientific evidence then available strongly suggested that household contact was not a factor in the spread of AIDS). A *Times* editorial then urged the federal government to spend more money on AIDS research.

The level of coverage in the *Los Angeles Times,* based on the same JAMA press release, was considerably more restrained, moving from 1 article in April, to 7 in May, 8 in June, 8 in July, 5 in August, and to 5 in September 1983.

The U.S. mass media reacted with sharply increased AIDS coverage in July 1985, once it was apparent that actor Rock Hudson was dying of AIDS. Hudson was not the only reason for the major increase in media attention given to AIDS at that time. During this same period, a study by Stanford University researchers warned of the exponential rate of spread of AIDS, *The New York Times* reported on a "wave of heterosexual anxiety in New York City," and the first reports of infants born with AIDS were released. The single most important influence that caused this dramatic increase in coverage was the public controversy about whether or not Ryan White, 13-year-old schoolboy who was diagnosed with AIDS, should be allowed to attend class with his schoolmates. *The New York Times* again greatly outpaced the *Los Angeles Times* in its number of articles about AIDS: 4 articles in June, to 16 in July, 46 in August, 72 in September, 77 in October, 60 in November, and settling at 51 in December. The *Los Angeles Times* had arrived at a comparable baseline by August; its monthly totals were 6 articles in June, 18 in July, 35 in August, 37 in September, 31 in October, 38 in November, and 32 in December.

The New York Times' coverage of AIDS was less consistent than coverage in either the *Los Angeles Times* or the *San Francisco Chronicle*. According to one analysis, alarmism and media sensationalism dominated national magazine coverage as well (Albert, 1989). Mass media coverage of AIDS may have been sensationalized, as well as slowed, by when and how the *Times* covered the issue.

Network Television and the Issue of AIDS

Network nightly newscasts show an over-time pattern of coverage of AIDS that is very similar to newspaper coverage. Our analysis of the television agenda for AIDS is based on data from the Vanderbilt Television News Archives, as well as a Vanderbilt Television News list of network AIDS special programs. From 1981 through December 1988, NBC carried 328 news stories, CBS aired 287 stories, and ABC broadcast 259 stories about AIDS. In addition, prior to January 1987, NBC had broadcast three AIDS specials (150 minutes), CBS two specials (90 minutes), and ABC devoted five segments of "Nightline" to AIDS (150 minutes) and broadcast one AIDS-related special (180 minutes). Only one of these 11 programs devoted to AIDS was broadcast prior to 1985 (PBS also broadcast two hour-long AIDS specials in 1984). Even more than newspapers, many television news stories about AIDS were unclear and confusing regarding how the disease is transmitted. Obfuscatory, euphemistic language ("exchange of bodily fluids'') did not tell audience members what they needed to know in order to avoid contracting the AIDS virus, and contributed to public over-reaction, such as firefighters refusing to help AIDS victims, and people not using public drinking fountains and restrooms.

With the exception of the *San Francisco Chronicle,* each of the newspapers and television networks that we studied displayed a very low level of AIDS coverage in 1984. Occasional blips of coverage were accorded to scientific reports about heterosexual transmission, blood transfusions, and saliva transmission. *Chronicle* coverage was dominated by the issue of closing the gay bathhouses in San Francisco, but this news was primarily treated as a local issue. Presidential primaries, a national election, and the 1984 Los Angeles Olympics pushed AIDS well down the national media agenda during 1984.

Both newspaper and television coverage of AIDS was more varied, less sensationalistic, and more patient-centered in 1990 than in the mid-1980s. Proportionately more stories about the need for compassion, caring, and respect of people with AIDS were written, and fewer inflammatory stories or stories about preliminary medical research as a ready cure for the disease are now broadcast or printed (Rogers et al., 1991). Many recent news stories are reassuring, as some network television news stories have tended to be all along (Colby & Cook, 1989).

Role of the Federal Government in Setting the Media Agenda

There was not an organized government response to AIDS in Washington, DC the way there was in San Francisco. The U.S. Public Health Service, the U.S. Department of Health and Human Services, and the National Institutes of Health did not respond to the presence of a new epidemic in a timely fashion (Shilts, 1987). For example, the National Institutes of Health did not call for applications for AIDS-related research until August 1982, over 1 year after the first alert by the Centers for Disease Control that an epidemic was underway.

Staff at the Centers for Disease Control tried to interest journalists in covering AIDS prior to 1985, but they were generally unsuccessful due to the perception that AIDS was a gay disease. The Centers for Disease Control did not, however, actively seek out media coverage for the epidemic as a means of informing and warning the public. Rather, they waited for journalists to come to them.

Although federal money was spent on AIDS epidemiology in fiscal year 1981, this funding was not a special appropriation, but a reallocation of money within the Centers for Disease Control. According to Congressional aides that we interviewed, official federal funding amounts for AIDS are difficult to interpret. For example, the federal government credits the National Institutes of Health with spending $3,355,000 on AIDS research in fiscal year 1982. The research that was conducted, however, dealt with virology problems that had little if anything to do with AIDS.

Early, relatively modest Congressional appropriations for AIDS were pushed through the House of Representatives and Senate by former Representative Phil Burton (D-San Francisco) and Representative Henry Waxman (D-Los Angeles). Both legislators represented large numbers of gay constituents. Representative Ted Weiss (D-New York City) also played an important role in investigating if and where, within the government, money for AIDS was being stalled. Gay staff members for these congressmen played crucial roles by first raising the issue of AIDS and doggedly sticking with the problem.

Throughout the 1980s, Congress approximately doubled Administration requests for AIDS funding each year. The White House was not committing much money to AIDS. Federal funding levels for AIDS research, education, and testing, which reached $2 billion in fiscal year 1990, might seem to be significant as preventive measures, until the costs of AIDS treatment are considered. The intermediate-level estimate for total U.S. medical costs due to AIDS from 1986 to 1991 is about $38 billion. The corresponding high estimate is $113 billion (Pascal, 1987).

A U.S. president can move the media on any particular issue. All he has to do is give a talk about it. President Reagan chose not to do so until May 1987, 72 months into the AIDS epidemic, a point at which 35,121 AIDS cases had been reported by the Centers for Disease Control. During the early years of the AIDS epidemic, the Reagan Administration generally ignored or downplayed the issue. In this period, the White House was mainly trying to cut the domestic budget, so as to help offset major increases for military defense and a trade deficit. In this context, AIDS represented a serious federal budget threat. Emergency AIDS money, like the funds earmarked for ongoing domestic programs, was subject to the Balanced Budget and Emergency Deficit Control Act of 1985, also known as the Gramm-Rudman-Hollings Act (Panem, 1988).

Certain federal officials, however, were very outspoken about the AIDS epidemic. Dr. C. Everett Koop, U.S. Surgeon General at the time, gave considerable attention to AIDS as a medical problem, and widely advocated using condoms for AIDS prevention. But Koop, as the nation's top medical officer, did not play an important role in shifting federal funding and personnel into AIDS research and education. In 1982, Dr. Edward Brandt, Assistant Secretary for Health, stated to the U.S. House of Representatives Subcommittee on Intergovernmental Relations and Human Resources that AIDS had been officially recognized by U.S. Secretary of Health and Human Services Margaret Heckler as "the Department's highest priority emergency health problem.'' Shortly thereafter, Secretary Heckler was "promoted" by the White House to the post of the U.S. ambassador to a small, distant nation.

The generally reluctant attitude of the Reagan Administration toward AIDS was in contrast to the basic public health strategy of throwing all available resources at an epidemic as quickly as possible. If AIDS had not first struck socially stigmatized segments of the U.S. population, the White House response might have been more proactive.

During the same years that the White House was ignoring the AIDS issue, it was pushing hard to raise the drug issue on the national news agenda. Former President Reagan and his wife Nancy (even more so) took a strong interest in the drug issue, and it climbed rapidly on the mass media agenda. The National Institute on Drug Abuse launched a major campaign in 1982, urging teen-agers to "Just say no" to drugs. The number of news stories about drugs increased sharply in the mid-1980s. But the real-world indicator of cocaine use in the U.S. had been leveling off since the 1970s, although a new drug, crack, was an increasing problem in certain urban areas (Danielian & Reese, 1989). White House anti-drug emphases were paralleled by dramatically increased mass media coverage of drug abuse, in spite of actual decreases in drug abuse (Bare, 1990). Clearly, the White House helped set the agenda for drugs (along with a key news event, the death of basketball star Len Bias in 1986), just as it did not set the agenda for AIDS.

INFLUENCES ON THE MEDIA'S NEWS AGENDA

The present analysis has shown that a variety of influences affected the importance of the issue of AIDS on the news agenda of mass media organizations. We found factors that made AIDS more important (i.e., which increased the number of stories about AIDS), and other factors that made the issue less important (i.e., which decreased the number of stories about AIDS) on news agendas.

In San Francisco, we found evidence of many more influences that pushed the issue of AIDS up news agendas than influences that pushed AIDS down news agendas. Influences that pushed AIDS up the local mass media news agenda included:

1. the highest rate of HIV infection of any North American city;
2. a strong commitment to the issue by several local journalists;
3. the well-organized networks of gays and medical professionals and their early resolve to help each other through forming and operating nonprofit groups;

4. the political importance and affluence of gays;
5. a mayor who was primed to acknowledge the salience of health issues;
6. the obstrusiveness of AIDS in San Francisco, where two of every five men were gay;
7. the savvy of a local television station in using the issue to satisfy the station's organizational goals;
8. controversy between conservative gays, who interpreted AIDS as a threat to their newly won personal rights, and liberal gays, who interpreted AIDS as a public health crisis; and
9. the liberal Democratic orientation of the Board of Supervisors, the members of which unanimously approved high levels of funding for AIDS education, epidemiology, research, testing, and treatment.

Factors that decreased the importance of AIDS on the local media agenda included:

1. public confusion about the disease; and
2. the lack of intermedia influence in San Francisco, where television stations and newspapers paid little attention to each other's coverage of AIDS and neither paid much attention to the extensive coverage given to the issue in the local gay news weeklies.

The mix of positive and negative influences on the importance of AIDS on the national media agenda was very different from that in San Francisco. In the United States, we found evidence that negative influences outweighed positive influences in determining the importance of the AIDS issue on the media agenda. Positive influences that pushed AIDS up the national mass media news agenda included:

1. the recurring and growing perception by editors in 1983, 1985, and 1987, that the issue was of interest and importance to mass audiences;
2. the mystery regarding means of HIV transmission;
3. the proclamations of Secretary Margaret Heckler and the forthrightness of Surgeon General C. Everett Koop, as the nation's top health officials;
4. the belated but concerted reporting about the political aspects of AIDS in *The New York Times*;
5. the commitment to the issue by a few journalists from influential media;

6. euphemistic language in mass media stories regarding the ways by which AIDS can be transmitted, which caused overreactions to the disease among many people; and

7. the scientific news agenda, which provided the mass media with a steady stream of research results about the disease.

Negative influences kept the AIDS issue a relatively unimportant media issue prior to June 1985. Negative factors included:

1. the slow-onset nature of the issue and its duration, neither of which are well-suited for garnering mass media attention;

2. the ideology dominant in the Reagan White House, in which military spending was increased at the expense of domestic programs, including health research and health care;

3. stigmatization of the segments in which the disease was initially concentrated;

4. editorial disinterest and homophobia, and personal factors at *The New York Times,* which served a nonagenda-setting role vis-à-vis other media organizations;

5. disorganization and competition among government bureaucracies;

6. the limited role the Centers for Disease Control in disseminating information to the U.S. public;

7. widespread confusion about AIDS transmission; and

8. the president's disinterest in the epidemic, in contrast to his declaration of war on a decreasing drug problem in the nation.

The present analysis shows that mass media organizations are far from autonomous actors in the determination of which issues become news. Media agendas, which are highly and positively correlated among mass media organizations, are determined by a host of endogenous and exogenous variables. Our analysis shows that for the issue of AIDS, whereas influences from within mass media organizations were important (both positively, such as a committed reporter at the *San Francisco Chronicle,* and negatively, such as a reluctant gatekeeper at *The New York Times*), outside variables (such as an efficacious network of gays and medical professionals, a very high rate of infection in San Francisco, and ideological opposition from a U.S. president) may have been more influential in determining the importance of AIDS on mass media news agendas. Thus, in the determination of what is news, mass media organizations are highly interdependent with their environment.

This interdependency is usually not considered in agenda-setting studies. Mass media news agendas are very determined by their environments, and other actors within those environments, so that (a) the same issue (b) studied over the same time period (c) but in different contexts, may reach a very different prominence due to the different environments within which organizations exist. The social and political environment of San Francisco, in which politics was dominated by efficacious gay groups, supported aggressive media coverage of the epidemic, although the content of that coverage was hotly debated. The tremendously larger context of the United States, in which gay groups were quite peripheral, did not encourage mass media organizations to pursue AIDS as an important topic until the threat of transmission was emphasized for heterosexuals. So attitudes of disinterest, homophobia, or indifference could effectively shape the response of the U.S. media until 1985. Research on media agenda-setting should conceptualize the output of mass media organizations as being closely responsive to the perceived attitudes and values held by efficacious groups of people within their relevant environment.

Both newspaper and television coverage of AIDS in the 1990s is a considerable improvement over the coverage of the 1980s. Editors and story assignment editors now acknowledge the importance of the AIDS issue, and its applicability to mass audiences. As AIDS has become legitimized as an important issue through extensive news and entertainment coverage, so too has the issue been routinized. Journalists are expected to write occasional AIDS stories. Governments are expected to continue certain levels of funding for AIDS education, testing, treatment, and research. The public is expected to take precautions against AIDS. Routinized issues, however, rarely satisfy the journalistic criteria for newsworthiness. The mass media have a short attention span. This characteristic is why, although news coverage of AIDS has increased from the early 1980s into the 1990s, this issue, like any issue, cannot remain continuously important on news agendas. Whereas the number of people afflicted with the disease continues to grow in the 1990s as epidemiologists have predicted, the pattern of mass media attention will appear cyclical in the 1990s, occupying alternately higher and lower positions on news agendas, just as it did in the 1980s. For any chronic disease, this pattern of a lack of correspondence between a real-world indicator, such as the number of afflicted persons, and media coverage measures, will hold due to the nature of news.

The present case informs our knowledge of agenda-setting theory in an important way besides demonstrating the cyclical nature of news issues and the lack of a strong positive correlation between amounts of issue coverage and real-world indicators of a problem. By focusing on the determinants of news coverage, we have found evidence of considerable interorganizational mass media interdependencies. That is, mass media organizations, whether conceptualized as operating within local interorganizational systems or national interorganizational and interinstitutional systems, are far from being alone in determining the importance of an issue on their news agendas. Interpersonal networks of concerned individuals, governments, community groups, scientific findings, and political leaders stand out in the present case as important determinants of news coverage about AIDS. Media organizations themselves played a relatively unimportant role as agenda-setters among themselves. One media organization played a key role in not setting the news agenda for the issue of AIDS. This result, that the most efficacious determinants of mass media news coverage were non-media sources, is an important finding for future research concerning influences on mass media news agendas.

REFERENCES

Albert, E. (1989). AIDS and the press: The creation and transformation of a social problem. In J. Best (Ed.), *Images of issues: Typifying contemporary social problems* (pp. 39–54). New York: Aldine De Gruyter.

Altman, D. (1986). *AIDS in the mind of America*. Garden City, NY: Anchor Press/Doubleday.

Arno, P. S. (1986). The nonprofit sector's response to the AIDS epidemic: Community-based services in San Francisco. *American Journal of Public Health, 76,* 1325–1330.

Atkin, C., & Arkin, E. B. (1990). Issues and initiatives in communicating health information to the public. In C. Atkin & L. Wallack (Eds.), *Mass communication and public health: Complexities and conflicts* (pp. 32–33). Newbury Park, CA: Sage.

Ball-Rokeach, S. J. (1985). The origins of individual media-system dependency: A sociological framework. *Communication Research, 12,* 485–510.

Bare, J. (1990). The war on drugs: A case study in opinion formation. *The Public Perspective: A Roper Center Review of Public Opinion and Polling, 2,* 29–31.

Brecher, E. M. (1988). Straight sex, AIDS, and the mixed-up press. *Columbia Journalism Review, 46,* 48–50.

Centers for Disease Control. (1988, April 4). *Centers for Disease Control surveillance report.* Atlanta, GA: U.S. AIDS Program, Center for Infectious Diseases.

Chaffee, S. (1980, June). Comments made as a discussant at the International Communication Association, Acapulco.

Check, W. A. (1987). Beyond the political model of reporting: Nonspecific symptoms in media communication about AIDS. *Review of Infectious Diseases, 9,* 987–1000.

Colby, D. C., & Cook, T. E. (1989, May). *The mass mediated epidemic: AIDS and television news 1981–1985.* Paper presented to the International Communication Association, San Francisco.

Danielian, L. H., & Reese, S. D. (1989). A closer look at intermedia influences on agenda-setting: The cocaine issue of 1986. In P. J. Shoemaker (Ed.), *Communication campaigns about drugs: Government, media, and the public* (pp. 47–65). Hillsdale, NJ: Lawrence Erlbaum Associates.

Dearing, J. W., & Rogers, E. M. (1988, May). *The agenda-setting process for the issue of AIDS.* Paper presented at the International Communication Association, New Orleans.

Dorfman, R. (1987, November 16). AIDS coverage: A mirror of society. *The Quill,* pp. 16–18.

Fitzgerald, F. (1986). *Cities on a hill.* New York: Simon & Schuster.

Hogan, M. A. (1988, February 21). In San Francisco, TV battles on the front lines against AIDS. *The New York Times,* p. H31.

Kinsella, J. (1988). Covering the plague years: Four approaches to the AIDS beat. *New England Journal of Public Policy, 4,* 465–474.

Kinsella, J. (1989). *Covering the plague: AIDS and the American media.* New Brunswick, NJ: Rutgers University Press.

Klaidman, S., & Beauchamp, T. (1987). *The virtuous journalist.* New York: Oxford University Press.

KPIX-TV. (1987). *AIDS Lifeline background.* San Francisco.

Kramer, S. D. (1988, March 12). The media and AIDS. *Editor & Publisher, 10,* pp. 10–11.

Lazarsfeld, P. F., & Merton, R. K. (1948). Mass communication, popular taste, and organized social action. In L. Bryson (Ed.), *The communication of ideas* (pp. 95–118). New York: Institute for Religious and Social Studies.

Linsky, M. (1986). *Impact: How the press affects Federal policymaking.* New York: Norton.

Mansbach, R. W., & Vasquez, J. A. (1981). *In search of theory: A new paradigm for global politics* (pp. 88–92). New York: Columbia University Press.

Meyer, P. (1990). News media responsiveness to public health. In C. Atkin & E. B. Arkin (Eds.), *Mass communication and public health: Complexities and conflicts* (pp. 52–59). Newbury Park, CA: Sage.

Panem, S. (1988). *The AIDS bureaucracy.* Cambridge, MA: Harvard University Press.

Pascal, A. (1987). *The cost of treating AIDS under Medicaid: 1986–1991, A Rand note.* Santa Monica, CA: Rand Corp.

Perrow, C., & Guillen, M. F. (1990). *The AIDS disaster.* New Haven, CT: Yale University Press.

Plough, A., & Krimsky, S. (1987). The emergence of risk communication studies: Social and political context. *Science, Technology, and Human Values, 12,* 4–10.

Qualter, T. H. (1985). *Opinion control in the democracies.* New York: St. Martin's Press.

Reese, S. (1991). Setting the media's agenda: A power balance perspective. In J. Anderson (Ed.), *Communication yearbook 14* (pp. 309–340). Newbury Park, CA: Sage.

Rogers, E. M., & Dearing, J. W. (1988). Agenda-setting research: Where has it been, where is it going? In J. A. Anderson (Ed.), *Communication yearbook 11* (pp. 555–594). Newbury Park, CA: Sage.

Rogers, E. M., Dearing, J. W., & Chang, S. (1991). AIDS in the 1980's: The agenda-setting process for a public issue. *Journalism Monographs, 126.*

Roper Center for Public Opinion Research. (1983–1990). As indicated by the responses of U.S. adults to over 500 survey questions about AIDS archived at the Roper Center from June 1983–December 1990.

San Francisco AIDS Foundation. (1987a). *Results from the fourth probability sample of an urban gay male community.* San Francisco: Author.

San Francisco AIDS Foundation. (1987b). *Media resource guide for AIDS information in San Francisco.* San Francisco: Author.

Scott, A. (1987, March 5). AIDS and the experts. *New Scientist,* pp. 50–52.

Shaw, D. (1987a, December 20). Coverage of AIDS story: A slow start. *Los Angeles Times,* p. A1.

Shaw, D. (1987b, December 21). Hudson brought AIDS coverage out of the closet. *Los Angeles Times,* p. A1.

Shilts, R. (1987). *And the band played on: Politics, people, and the AIDS epidemic.* New York: St. Martin's Press.

Shoemaker, P. J., & Reese, S. (1991). *Mediating the message.* New York: Longman.

Shoemaker, P. J., with Mayfield, E. K. (1987). Building a theory of news content: A synthesis of current approaches. *Journalism Monographs, 103.*

Singer, E., & Rogers, T. F. (1987). Public opinion and AIDS. *AIDS and Public Policy Journal, 1,* 8–13.

Singer, E., Rogers, T. F., & Corcoran, M. (1987). The polls: A report: AIDS. *Public Opinion Quarterly, 51,* 580–595.

Winsten, J. A. (1985). Science and the media: The boundaries of truth. *Health Affairs, 4,* 5–23.

CHAPTER TEN

AIDS, Medicalization, and the News Media

Matthew P. McAllister
*Virginia Polytechnic Institute
and State University*

Health communication is one area of specialization that has achieved an important level of prominence in communication scholarship within the last 5 years. There exists now a journal devoted solely to the topic, *Health Communication*. The International Communication Association has a Health Communication Division, and the association's 41st annual conference had as its theme "Communication and Health." A trip to the library reveals such recent academic books as *Communicating with Medical Patients* (Stewart & Roter, 1989) and *Communication and Medical Practice* (Silverman, 1988). This academic interest in health communication has been fueled by, among other factors, the devastating existence of Acquired Immune Deficiency Syndrome and the contribution communication studies can make to the social understanding of the condition.

Yet the bulk of this health communication research, including the research focusing on AIDS issues, generally comes out of one paradigm of communication research: the paradigm that embraces applied and administrative research. In discussing an area related to health communication—scholarly writing about the relationships between science and the media—Dornan (1990) argued that such writing is characterized by a celebration of scientific institutions and the scientific method. Health communication may be described in a similar fashion. Traditionally, health communication scholarship has taken as its basic assumptions the same assumptions held by mainstream Western medicine: (a) The goals of the medical profession are the only goals of good health; (b) physician's opinions and recommendations are to be accepted by patients and the general public, and when they are not accepted something needs to be done to change the patients and public; and (c) medicine is an apolitical entity, existing only to improve the health of citizens.

Although we learn much from research done in this tradition, no one paradigm may answer all questions. For example, illness as a medical and social phenomenon involves social power. This statement is especially true of AIDS, as was made clear very early in its history: how AIDS is discussed, how resources are allocated, who are defined as in the "risk groups," and who make the decisions about AIDS highlight the inseparable connection between AIDS and power in society. AIDS is the most explicitly politicized of medical conditions. Health communication as a well-rounded academic specialization, then, should include not just research that seeks to improve the efficiency of doctor–patient relationships or mass-mediated health campaigns, but also research that incorporates critical theory: research that attempts to explain and understand the political aspects of illness and the role communication plays.

The objective of this chapter is to explore the possible contribution of one critical approach toward medicine to the understanding of how the news media have constructed the AIDS phenomenon. This approach is called *medicalization,* which highlights the expansive and political nature of medicine. As such, the chapter (a) reviews the medicalization literature, and its two main themes, the medicalization of everyday life and medicine as an institution for social control; (b) explicates connections between medicalization and the news media, arguing that news is especially susceptible to medicalized world views; and (c) argues for the news media's potential for presenting both an uncritical acceptance of medicalized perspectives of AIDS, as well as occasional criticism of such perspectives.

THE MEDICALIZATION OF SOCIETY

Contributions to the theory of medicalization come from many different academic disciplines, including traditional sociology (Parsons, 1951), medical sociology (Zola, 1972), bioethics (Engelhardt, 1986), psychiatry (Szasz, 1961, 1970), feminism (Ehrenreich & English, 1978; Treichler, 1990), critical history (Foucault, 1975, 1977), Marxism (Navarro, 1975), philosophy of technology (Illich, 1976), gay studies (Bayer, 1981), and literary criticism (Sontag, 1979, 1988). This theory attempts to understand and explain the expansion of the medical institution or a medical ideology as forms of cultural authority, especially when such medical authority is used to explain or control different aspects of life.

Two major themes, or areas of focus, are prevalent in the medicalization literature. These themes are (a) the medicalization of everyday life and (b) the medicalization of deviance, with the latter's concentration on medicine as a form of social control. It should be remembered that although for purposes of clarity these two themes are discussed separately, they are interrelated, and many theorists concentrate on both aspects of medicalization.

The Medicalization of Everyday Life: Two Perspectives

The most encompassing theme of the medicalization literature is the increasing role of medicine in our lives. As one scholar described this process:

> Medicine medicalizes reality. It creates a world. It translates sets of problems into its own terms. Medicine molds the ways in which the world of experience takes shape; it conditions reality for us. The difficulties people have are then appreciated as illness, diseases, deformities, and medical abnormalities, rather than as innocent vexations, normal pains, or possession by the devil. (Engelhardt, 1986, p. 157)

Several researchers have looked into the different levels of medicalization in our society, and the phenomenon's pervasiveness. Basically, however, the perspectives of two writers, Irving Kenneth Zola and Ivan Illich, encompass most of the issues involved with how our everyday lives are medicalized.

Zola (1972), for example, presented four different ways in which the medicalization of society occurs. The first way is in the ever increasing realm of health-related items and the emphasis on the use of a multicausal view of disease in mainstream medicine. When visiting physicians, patients must reveal to the physicians more and more about their lives. This way of medicalizing life also points to what has been called *healthism*, where diet, lifestyle, and employment become thought of purely in terms of health, and personal changes are made in these areas in the name of health (Crawford, 1980). The second level of medicalization for Zola is achieved when the medical profession retains absolute control over certain techniques and procedures. This aspect includes not only the allocation of drugs and the use of surgery, but also professional autonomy from outside control and the specialized language used by medical professionals. Zola's third point is that medicalization increases when the medical profession retains absolute control over certain "taboo" areas of society. Now aging, drug addiction, and pregnancy are all considered to be under the nearly exclusive purview of medicine. The physician becomes a main solver of social and personal problems. An elaboration of this third point is presented by Ruzek (1978), who argued that several crucial life events of women, such as pregnancy, childbirth, and menopause, have been co-opted by medical control. The final process is through what Zola called "the expansion of what in medicine is deemed relevant to the good practice of life" (p. 496). This last point is perhaps most relevant to communication, in that it indicates the power of evoking medicalized rhetoric to increase the credibility of proposals, as well as the health connections made to such institutions as the media, schools, and the workplace. The recent work of Treichler (1987, 1988) points to the potential power of medicalized language in AIDS discourse.

To summarize Zola's four perspectives, the medicalization of everyday life involves two different types of medical expansion (Getz & Hawkins, 1979). The first type is an expansion of the authority of the medical profession: the power of health-care physicians and medical researchers. Society recognizes "medical professional authority" when it dictates, "physicians have the authority to perform this activity." The second type is an expansion of the medical model. The medical model, or a medical ideology, is a model that advocates that problems of human existence are best solved by treating individuals separately and "curing" them. Medicalization occurs, then, when this medical perspective (focusing on the individual as a problem-solving strategy) is applied to different areas of life. Thus, "medical ideological authority" is granted when society says, "this phenomenon is best understood as individual illness." This second type of medicalization, of course, may be wielded by doctors, but also by nonmedical personnel. Thus, although some critics, such as Fox (1977), claim that medicalization is decreasing because of the emergence of nonprofessions in medicine, like nurse practitioners and physician assistants, other writers answer that Fox is only addressing medical professional authority, and true demedicalization only occurs when both medical professional authority and medical ideological authority decreases (Conrad, 1980).

The second perspective of the medicalization of everyday life comes from the most read and controversial theorist of medicalization, Ivan Illich, a former Catholic priest who passionately writes about the inherent danger of corrupted and overextended technology to the autonomy of the human spirit. Illich (1976) attacked the medical industry as being guilty of such an overextension in his book *Medical Nemesis*. Highlighting the *consequences* of the medicalization of everyday life, Illich claimed that medicine has become so technological in its orientation, and so expansive in its reach, that this institution, rather than being a healer, has itself created three new levels of disease, or iatrogenic ailments. The first level he delineated as clinical iatrogenesis, in which the specific techniques and procedures used by medicine cause more physical illness than they cure. Thus, examples of clinical iatrogenesis would include the side effects of drugs and radiation treatments, and advancement of illness caused when patients are lost in the shuffle of medical specialization. The second form of iatrogenesis is social, in which health-care treatment becomes a commodity, and even birth and death are profit-generating avenues. Finally, at the deepest level of corruption is cultural iatrogenesis. Illich argued that human life has become so medicalized that we can no longer deal with suffering, pain, death, and even health with any degree of autonomy. As a culture, our coping methods have been replaced by medical industrialization. Because of this, "pain thus turns into a demand for more drugs, hospitals, medical services, and other outputs of corporate, impersonal care and into political support for further corporate growth no matter what its human, social, or economic cost" (p. 132). For Illich, then, the solution to medicalization is self-help: the development of technologies that encourage autonomy and less dependence on health professionals. Although some scholars, most notably Navarro (1975), criticize Illich for not paying sufficient attention to the role of economics and class biases in medicalization, they for the most part agree with Illich's interpretation of its overwhelmingly negative consequences.

In fact, Illich is not the only theorist who highlights the destructive results of medicalization. Most medicalization theorists emphasize that medicine's expansion into everyday life does not occur neutrally. Such expansion has social and political consequences: consequences that may reinforce already existing power inequalities. In accordance with this, one other theme dominant in the literature is the medicalization of deviance: medicalization as a form of social control.

The Medicalization of Deviance

Conrad and Schneider (1980) proposed that the treatment and rhetoric of deviance in our society has to some degree "evolved" over the centuries. Originally deviance was under the purview of religion: Deviance was looked upon and discussed as sinful, and corrected accordingly. Later, as the state became more powerful, the society's definition of deviant behavior changed, and matters of law and justice were more relevant: Deviance was seen as crime. Finally, in the most "modern" stages of deviance definition, the occurrence is viewed in medical terms: The deviance is viewed as a manifestation of illness. Thus alcoholism, insanity, homosexuality, and drug addiction have all passed through these three basic stages (although they do overlap to a large degree at times).

This medicalization of deviance is beneficial to the dominant institutions of society: The classification of an illness is not clearly or simply biomedical in all cases, and not "objective," but rather mirrors social organization and the dominant ideology. Several examples illustrate how disease classification reflects dominant viewpoints and "social expectations." Blacks in the 19th century, for instance, were vulnerable to health designations that, in retrospect, were devices for social control. Szasz (1970) noted that Dr. Benjamin Rush, the "father of American psychiatry," believed Blacks to be afflicted with the illness "Negritude," a genetic form of mild leprosy that caused a darkening of the skin. As the medical critic pointed out, "With this theory, Rush made the Negro a medically safe domestic, while at the same time called for the sexual segregation of a carrier of a dread hereditary disease" (p. 155). Perhaps more blatant is an example told by Conrad and Schneider (1980). They related the story of an American physician in the South who, in 1851, published an article in an influential health journal that described "drapetomania," a disease that only afflicted Black slaves and was manifested by the behavior of trying to escape from the plantations and the slave's master.

Women, also, have been the subjects of medicalization for the purposes of social control. For example, although there was little, if any, medical evidence that the accepted treatment made women more biomedically healthy (Ehrenreich & English, 1978), some writers have speculated that the sexual surgery of over 150,000 women (Barker-Benfield, 1978) during the 19th century was the result of male anxiety over women's growing power in society (Barker-Benfield, 1978). As Ehrenreich and English (1978) argued, gynecological surgery was the "solution" for many behaviors; "promiscuity, dancing in hot rooms, and subjection to an overly romantic husband were given as the origins of illness, along with too much reading, too much seriousness or ambition, and worrying" (p. 44).

Nor is the social control aspect of medicine exclusively a 19th-century phenomenon. Szasz (1970) noted that many German psychiatrists contributed to the development of gas chambers in Nazi Germany and the selection of the mentally ill as the first victims; medical rationales for the Holocaust were also offered by some physicians. More recently, Katz and Abel (1984) discussed how psychiatrists in the Soviet Union applied a "schizophrenic" label to dissident behavior and, in the United States, how some of the urban protests and violent outbreaks during the late 1960s could perhaps be explained by "organic brain dysfunction," according to two noted neurosurgeons and a neuropsychiatrist in an infamous letter to the *Journal of the American Medical Association* (Mark, Sweet, & Ervin, 1967, p. 217).

As discussed at the beginning of this chapter, early studies of the social control aspects of medicine focused on psychiatry and mental institutions. Szasz, for example, noted in 1961 the social influences of psychiatric labeling, and the fact that the study of power relationships in the labeling process is important in completely understanding "the myth of mental illness." Szasz believed, in the case of mental illness, the labels were not scientifically rational, but in fact were socially constructed and not to the benefit of those labeled. Similarly, Goffman's (1961) book *Asylums* questioned the objectivity of the medical model in the mental institutional setting.

Other researchers began to note the ideological aspects not only of psychiatry and psychology, but of more "objective" medicine as well. The first scholar to use the term *medicalization of deviance* was Jesse Pitts in the *International Encyclopedia of the Social Sciences* in 1968. Pitts expanded on Talcott Parsons' (1951) notion of the sick role, and discussed the effectiveness of medicine not simply to control biomedical deviance (such as catching a cold), but also social deviance as well. Pitts described the efficiency of medicine as social control: "if the culprit pleads illness, he thereby certifies his commitment to the dominant values and institutionalized norms and implies that, when restored to health, he will conform . . ." (p. 391). Medical control is especially efficient because it *de*politicizes any issues that the deviant raises—the deviant is, after all, sick—and it presents an image of compassion for the deviant, while also being "value-free" and politically neutral.

In addition, Zola (1972) pointed to the definition of societal problems that medicalization encourages. If an individual is ill, according to the traditional medical model, you treat the individual, either by preventative or curative means. If social conditions are the "cause" of the illness, traditional medical ideology gives social conditions no attention, focusing instead on changing the individual: More macro forms of intervention are ignored (Zola, 1972). So, although some argue that medicalization is the most humane mechanism for social control (Knowles, 1977), it is also one of the most subtle and effective for the status quo.

In the aforementioned instances, deviance is labeled as illness. Others have taken Parsons' sick role a step further by arguing that many times illness may be labeled as social deviance. For example, the connection between dominant norms and groups, on the one hand, and illness, on the other, is strengthened by Sontag (1979) in her much-quoted *Illness as Metaphor*. The social connotations of certain illnesses—their cultural metaphor—may lead to a "blaming of the victim." Socially undesirable attributes, rather than being defined as an illness in and of themselves, are defined as the causes of illness. Thus, two illustrations of a "blame the victim" medicalized social control are Western views of tuberculosis and cancer. As Sontag pointed out, "The tubercular could be an outlaw or a misfit; the cancer personality is regarded more simply, and with condescension, as one of life's losers" (p. 55). And not only may psychological characteristics be defined as illness-causing; so may demographic characteristics. Pence (1989) observed that the stereotypes of the drunken Irish, the lazy Blacks and the unclean poor were often used to explain outbreaks of cholera. As is discussed later, this Sontagian perspective on illness has been applied to discourse about AIDS by several writers.

Most medicalization theorists argue that the process is increasing in our society because of an expansion of medical ideology, if not the actual medical profession. With increasing government involvement in medicine (in the form of diagnostic related groups), the increased role of private business interests (for-profit medical organizations are becoming more prevalent), increased consumer involvement in health treatment, as well as the pervasiveness of AIDS issues, the application of the medical model is expanding into other sectors of society, even while, as Fox (1977) suggested, the medical profession itself may be losing influence over certain sectors. In other words, despite these trends leading to a potential "crisis of medical [professional] authority" (Fox, 1988), the same trends may lead to an expansion of medical ideological authority. As this expansion increases, the study of medicalization will become more and more vital.

Recently, in fact, other medicalization theorists have looked at the intrusion of medicine into many different aspects of modern life: religion (Robbins & Anthony, 1982); management/labor relations (Roman, 1980); and current women/power relations (Calnan, 1984; Riessman, 1983), including childbirth (Treichler, 1990), among others. Yet very little work has concentrated on the role of the news media in the medicalization process. The following section attempts to lay some basic groundwork for this area.

MEDICALIZATION AND NEWS MEDIA STUDIES

Because one thesis of medicalization is that medicine expands its purview throughout society, and one way medicalization occurs is through the use of medicalized language, it is surprising that more explicit connections between the theory of medicalization and the mass media (especially the news media—society's disseminator of information) have not been made. Those who have touched upon the role of the news in medicalization highlight the willingness of the press to accept medicalized perspectives. Clarke (1984) discussed the use of medicalized portrayals of deviance in news, and argued that medicalized explanations have found prominence in news stories about women's liberation, draft resisters, and issues of race, ethnicity, and religious and sexual orientation. Likewise, Karpf (1988) very briefly discussed the acceptance of medicalized sources and perspectives in the electronic media, arguing that broadcasting's need for quick explanations and authoritative sources makes physicians the perfect television news expert.

In fact, there are structural incentives that encourage all mainstream news media to be accepting of medicalized discourse. At least three aspects of news would seem to warn of the dangers of medicalization in the news media: (a) the concordance between the news value of objectivity and medicalized perspectives, (b) the dependence of journalists on medical sources, and (c) the rhetorical necessities of journalism.

News Objectivity and Medicalization

Sigal (1973), Tuchman (1978), Carey (1987), and Bennett (1988) all highlighted how the empirical tradition of news (verifiable objectivity) limits what it may say on a routine basis. Because news must be "objective," it must be grounded in the observable and in the factual. Thus, explanations in news tend to be at the lowest level of abstraction: that of personalized motives (Carey, 1987). On the other hand, broad sociological explanations do not fit in well with the Five-W-and-H format (addressing in the lead paragraphs the Who, What, Where, When, Why, and How of the story), and tend to take a back seat to more concrete frameworks: Frameworks that, although verifiable and observable, are also historically and sociologically contextless (see Bennett, 1988, pp. 44–51 for a more detailed explanation of how journalistic norm of objectivity leads to "fragmented," contextless news).

Viewing the structure of news in this manner may reveal structural biases toward the presentation of medicalized perspectives and stories. The medical model of treatment, with its usually quick, empirical, individual focus, fits in very nicely with professional news value of objectivity (Karpf, 1988). Alternatively, fundamental critiques of medical ideological authority, critiques that would require discussions of enduring conditions and notions of societal power, do not fit easily into a "Five-W-and-H" format.

Besides potentially legitimating and depoliticizing medicine, the reciprocity of objectivity in news with the medical model may have another unfortunate consequence. By focusing explanations on the individual, news could reinforce the social stigma of those who are sick. That is, news could reinforce the acceptance of "illness as metaphor" frameworks (Sontag, 1979). News could subtly blame certain sick people for their illness, especially if these people are somehow "deviant" in their behavior or social persona. The undesirable social characteristics of the individual might be implied in news as causing their illness. Thus, the personal explanation, a characteristic of news, fits in quite well with a "blaming of the victim" perspective. Several critics, among them Altman (1986), Watney (1986, 1987), and Treichler (1987, 1988), have argued that news coverage of people living with AIDS is characterized by this perspective, as is developed later.

Journalists and Medical Sources

A second factor that would point to an acceptance of medicalization by mainstream newspapers is the dependent relationships that journalists have on medical sources. Sources for biomedical stories are especially revered by journalists because of the social "awe" for science and the technical nature of research. Kinsella (1989) called this the "Gee Whiz" attitude of journalists toward science and medicine. So, for example, medical journals are important in medical news, becoming nearly unquestioned as sources, and publishers of medical journals realize the nature of this relationship. As Karpf (1988) explained, prestigious medical journals send major news outlets early copies of each issue, requiring that the newspaper delay publication of any stories based on the issue until the official publication of the issue. This allows journalists the time to prepare their stories so that the news stories and the journal issue may be published on the same date.

Research indicates that mainstream medicine does indeed "set the agenda" for medical news. One study found the three journals *Nature, Science,* and *Lancet* provided the most information to two BBC radio broadcasts (cited in Cronholm & Sandell, 1981). Another study found that from January 1984 to April 1988 the *New England Journal of Medicine* was cited 500 times by major U.S. print media, nearly twice as much as any other science or medically oriented publication (*Journal of the American Medical Association* was second with 263 cites) (cited in Kinsella, 1989). Finally, Fisher, Gandy, and Janus (1981) found an overwhelming use of the mainstream medical establishment as the source for health stories appearing between 1959 and 1974 in three popular magazines. So there has been a traditional dependence on medical sources for medical news. But other, more recent, factors are strengthening the ability of medicine to influence news. Medical professional authority may be finding an even firmer acceptance in news with recent developments.

First of all is the development of the "health beat" reporter. This position has been created in many newspapers (including *The New York Times,* with its hiring of a medical doctor, Lawrence K. Altman, as its medical reporter) to increase their coverage of medical issues. The creation of such a position allows medicine to have a guaranteed, routinized conduit through which medical stories are generated. It also guarantees that reporters interact with certain health and medical authorities on a regular basis. A continual relationship (a relationship characteristic of beat reporting) is created. Gans (1979) noted that beat reporters, because of their continuing relationships with certain sources, may feel they must keep their sources happy. Health beat reporters, then, become obligated to give more favorable coverage to health-care organizations than existed in the past because of the development of this new reporter–source relationship.

Additionally, as more news outlets establish health beat positions, there is the possibility for the development of a health "pack": a small number of health reporters who become acquainted with each other and begin to cooperate during the news gathering process (see Dunwoody, 1980; and Bennett, 1988, pp. 115–116 for discussions of pack reporting). As Dunwoody pointed out, the development of a pack makes particular sense on highly technical beats, such as science or health. The development of a pack offers advantages in the news gathering process, such as offering reporters time saving techniques (through the sharing of notes) and a certain leverage over sources (as reporters may "team up" on uncooperative sources during press conferences), but there are some disadvantages that would seem to encourage medicalized reporting.

As previous research has noted (Bennett, 1988; Dunwoody, 1980), one characteristic to pack reporting is the pressure to conform in reporting. Thus, pack reporters tend to write stories on the same topics, from the same perspectives, using the same sources. Beat news stories written by different journalists for different news organizations tend to be homogeneous. This characteristic, however, would not necessarily lead to medicalized news, except when combined with a second potential disadvantage. Because health and medical news is highly technical, reporters on the pack would tend to look to the most experienced and knowledgeable reporters to confirm interpretations and to "set the agenda" for what is important. To reiterate a point made earlier, many of the most knowledgeable journalists on the health beat are medically trained (such as Altman of *The New York Times*). Therefore, journalists who already subscribe to a medical perspective may be the ones most influential in the pack. Homogeneous news may become medicalized news. Indeed, Pfund and Hofstadter (1981) pointed out that news coverage of biomedical research such as recombinant DNA is very homogeneous, often reflecting the point of view of large research organizations and virtually ignoring dissident views.

In addition to the creation of the health beat and health pack, the journalist–medical source dependence is perpetuated by the increased public relations activities of medical organizations. This includes both biomedical research organizations (as noted by Gandy, 1982; Karpf, 1988; Nelkin, 1985, 1987; Winsten, 1985), and local hospitals and health-care organizations (Folland, 1985) looking to become more media-wise in an uncertain market. News sources most beneficial to journalists—the sources most used by journalists—are those who are accessible, reliable, and skilled in news management. Large health-care organizations are quickly becoming those types of sources. They are becoming more skilled at placing stories in the news. Given all of these factors surrounding the medical source–journalist relationship (the traditional dependence, the health beat influence, and the increased media activity), what are some results of the increased dependence on medical sources by journalists? In fact, these factors could lead to an increase not just in the use of both medical professional authority in news, but also in the use of medical ideological authority as well.

As Sigal (1973) argued, one process that is involved in writing a news story is role-playing: Journalists must adopt, at least temporarily, the perspectives of their sources (especially their major sources) in order to completely understand that sources' viewpoints and communicate those viewpoints to a readership. According to Sigal:

> Without role-taking, without putting [him or herself] in official's shoes, a reporter might find it somewhat harder to anticipate the outcomes of controversies, or even to understand what a source's comments mean. Yet repeated role-taking may lead [him/her] to adopt the official's perspective on issues. The line between role-taking and absorption is a thin one indeed. (p. 47)

It follows that this process operates when sources are medical sources. In fact, because of the technical and professional nature of medicine, the danger is even greater that journalists must essentially co-opt themselves to medical sources. As medical sources make themselves more available for stories, more role-playing takes place. Eventually, then, the medical professional authority exercised because of source dependence may become a medical ideological authority: Journalists adopt the basic framework of their medical sources when writing their stories. This danger may be especially a factor when only medical sources are used in a story. The medical model eventually may overwhelm other interpretive frameworks that the health beat reporter may have applied.

A second related effect of medical source dependence is that it may lead to a lack of criticism of medicine in news. For example, as noted earlier prestigious medical journals play a large role in setting the agenda for medical research news coverage. Yet the level of criticism of medicine and science is superficial. By generating news stories from medical journals, editors and news writers are depending on a (basically) celebratory vehicle as their primary source (Karpf, 1988). Likewise, those most efficacious for news are those most skilled at news management: those with the resources to hire skilled public and media relations experts either to talk to news directly, or to teach others to talk to news. Those with alternative or dissenting medical opinions may not be firmly placed in the medical establishment, and thus may not have access to such news management resources. Referring back to the findings of Pfund and Hofstadter (1981), the increase in media relations activity in medicine may further dichotomize medicine into loud dominant voices, and quiet oppositional voices.

Finally, the dependence on dominant medical sources could also lead to the further increase of the medicalization of everyday life, where medical professional authority and medical ideological authority become applied to nonbiomedical areas. As medical sources become available, it could be the case that journalists will use these sources for opinions about other areas outside of their traditional purview. A study by Dunwoody and Ryan (1987), for example, surveyed scientists who had been used as sources by the news media. Of this sample, 61% stated that at least a portion of the news interview had dealt with topics outside of their areas of research expertise. Given the results of the Dunwoody and Ryan study, as well as the number of scholars who have written about medicalization, it seems reasonable to expect such an expansion of authority by the press of medical researchers as well.

Medicalization and the Rhetorical Necessity of News

Thus far two news production factors that would seem to encourage the placement of medicalized authority in the news media have been discussed: objectivity and source dependence. One last factor occurs at the moment of the construction of the news story. Hall, Critcher, Jefferson, Clarke, and Roberts (1978) argued that this moment involves a negotiation process in which the journalist considers the needs of his or her audience, writing the story so that comprehension will be maximized for this assumed audience. Rhetorically, the journalist must take unfamiliar events and facts and construct them in such a way that they become familiar and understandable to the reader. This process of making the strange familiar, a process that occurs for both the journalist and the journalist's audience, may also lead to medicalization.

Given this rhetorical purpose of journalism, the communication of scientific research to a mass audience involves a dilemma. Because the construction of scientific research, including biomedical research, is a complicated process, how does the journalist boil down the process in such a way that the audience will understand the research? One way is to remove the complications. As Nelkin (1987) explained, an important tool in creating understanding is the metaphor, a tool that simplifies complex ideas. Especially in science and medical news, metaphorical language is important in communicating complex and technical ideas to a mass audience.

But metaphors, in addition to creating understanding, also transform ideas. When writers compare one thing to another, they are implying that the two share common characteristics. Thus, writers highlight certain characteristics with metaphors, and de-emphasize others. The choice of descriptive wordings, Nelkin continued, "can trivialize an event or render it important; marginalize some groups, empower others; define an issue as a problem or reduce it to a routine" (p. 11).

Metaphors, then, are powerful devices that journalists use to make the scientific process—a strange and unfamiliar process—familiar to themselves and their audiences. Metaphors contribute to how people understand science, and react to it. Some metaphors are more positive than others, and some imply that further action is needed:

> When high technology is associated with "frontiers" that are maintained through "battles" or "struggles," the imagery of war implies that the experts should not be questioned, that new technologies must go forward and that limits are inappropriate. (Nelkin, 1987, p. 81)

The point is that certain metaphors are more beneficial to dominant scientific and medical powers than others. If medical organizations are becoming more media wise, then surely they will take advantage of the journalist's need for metaphorical understanding by supplying the metaphors themselves. Because journalists must make the medically strange familiar for themselves and their audiences, this—coupled with the increased media activity by medical organizations—could lead to the placing of more favorable medical metaphors in news.

An additional point is involved with the process of making the strange familiar. Journalists, occasionally, will be forced to write about groups that they find so strange they cannot identify with. The dilemma of source role-playing was mentioned earlier. Radical groups, groups of oppositional or alternative understandings, may not fit neatly in a journalist's cognitive frame, especially if the group questions institutions that the journalist fundamentally believes in. How, then, does the journalist attempt to understand such groups, and communicate this understanding to a mass audience?

With the increased availability of medical sources, this dilemma might be solved for the journalist: "frame" the deviants in a medical model. More accessibility by medical sources for opinions of news events, when coupled with a journalistic inclination to expand the purview of scientific authority (Dunwoody & Ryan, 1987), could lead to a "medicalization" of such groups. Furthermore, the fact that this framing is viewed by many in society as humane (at least compared to a criminal frame) would seem to encourage this tendency: The deviant is not weird, the deviant is sick. But despite the intentions of the journalist, as discussed earlier such a medical frame delegitimizes and depoliticizes issues raised by the person defined as deviant.

Possibilities for Demedicalization in News

Such is the picture presented of the mainstream newspapers' acceptance of medicine: The three factors of objectivity, source dependence, and making the strange familiar would seem to overwhelmingly point to strong "relations of reciprocity" with medicine and newspapers. But there are possibilities for exceptions to this reciprocity. Thus, for example, such scholars as Gans (1979) and Shoemaker (1987) imply that the press' constant, economically oriented need to produce the novel and the exciting may lead to occasional criticism of fundamental institutions, including medicine. Given the news value of progressive reform, if certain medical organizations or individuals break basic tenets of medicine, the degree of criticism leveled at them could be formidable.

Also, if medical sources gain power as news sources, this could lead to another avenue of criticism of the medical institution, at least on some levels. Two scholars, Molotch and Lester (1974), noted that most news consists of what they called "routines," or self-serving events promoted by elite powers. However, also found in news are "accidents" (inadvertent occurrences, embarrassing for a social elite, that are publicized by other, antagonistic, social elites, like the incident at Three Mile Island), and/or "scandals" (planned, but covert, occurrences of a social elite, that are publicized by other social elites, such as Watergate). The authors wrote that accidents and scandals, basically publicized conflicts between elites, perhaps facilitated by their role as news sources, can help reveal society's underlying power structure by providing a glimpse into that structure's workings. If medical sources begin using news to advance their own agendas, this could lead to the occasional medical "accident" or "scandal" in the news.

Despite the possibility for such leaks, the production process of mainstream news structures an overall acceptance of medicalized authority. But how does this perspective help us to understand news coverage of AIDS? The next section reviews this issue.

AIDS, MEDICALIZATION, AND THE NEWS

Mainstream news portrayals of AIDS have been the subject of articles in the areas of media studies, health studies, and gay studies, among others. The role of the mainstream news media is seen as crucial in society's understanding of AIDS. Indeed, the agenda-setting influence of American media coverage of AIDS may be global (Altman, 1986). A review of the literature reveals two characteristics of AIDS news coverage that highlight the relationship between news, AIDS, and medicalization: (a) the stigmatization of certain groups in AIDS news coverage, and (b) a dependence on medicine in such coverage.

The Stigmatization of Perceived Risk Groups in the News

As discussed earlier, Sontag (1979) observed how in our culture certain illnesses carry meanings other than biomedical, and these nonbiomedical meanings may become so strong that an ill person becomes almost exclusively labeled and defined as a person with that specific illness. The illness, because of its nonbiomedical connotations, becomes a metaphor for characteristics attributed to that person. Several scholars (Altman, 1986; Brandt, 1988; Hughey, Norton, & Sullivan, 1986; Sontag, 1988; Treichler, 1987) have noted that one way AIDS has been "medicalized" is through the invention of nonbiomedical cultural meanings for AIDS, and the inseparable link that has been made between certain demographic groups and AIDS. Thus, these cultural meanings become associated with the groups as well. AIDS, then, becomes a part of these groups' identity: It becomes a metaphor for attributed personal characteristics of members of these groups. Many scholars who have written about early AIDS coverage note that, when the press did discuss AIDS, it was in a way that perpetuated the AIDS-as-group-metaphor process (Albert, 1986a, 1986b; Altman, 1986; Baker, 1986; Karpf, 1988; Patton, 1985; Schwartz, 1984; Seidman, 1988; Treichler, 1987, 1988; Watney, 1986, 1987). AIDS-as-a-group-metaphor was established in three ways: the strong early association in news coverage of the gay lifestyle with AIDS; the emphasis on risk group's "deviant" properties; and the rhetorical blockage of identification with those afflicted by AIDS.

Albert (1986b) noted that when society discussed AIDS, the binding of the stereotypical image of a "gay lifestyle" with AIDS became unbreakable. Early media coverage contributed greatly to this linkage. Headlines from 1982 AIDS stories reveal the strong association made between gay lifestyles and the newly discovered condition: from *New York Magazine,* readers found "The Gay Plague" (Albert, 1986a); from the Philadelphia

Daily News there was "Gay Plague Baffling Medical Detectives"; from *The Saturday Evening Post* there appeared "Being Gay Is a Health Hazard"; and from the Toronto *Star* there was "Gay Plague Has Arrived in Canada" (the latter three cited in Altman, 1986). An exclusive relationship was presented between gays and AIDS despite the fact that as early as August 1981 heterosexuals were being reported by the Centers for Disease Control (CDC) as experiencing immune deficiency. Why, then, the early linking?

One reason may be the lack of information about the condition. Albert (1986a) argued that, "Lacking information on 'what' the sufferers had, 'who' they were became grist for the mill" (p. 145). Also, given the news media's dependence on medical sources, it could be that the nature of the medical sources for early AIDS stories influenced the strength of the gay/AIDS connection. The CDC was the nearly exclusive source for stories in 1981 and 1982, and given the epidemiological emphasis of that organization, it tended to stress the "who" more than anything else (Albert, 1986a). A third reason was that many of the medical researchers themselves ignored exceptions to the accepted AIDS/gay epidemiological theories and thus when these researchers were used as sources the exceptions are not discussed. For example, one 1982 study was entitled "Gay-Related Immunodeficiency (GRID) Syndrome: Clinical and Autopsy Observations." The GRID label was used in this title even though 2 of the 10 subjects in the study were exclusively heterosexual (Oppenheimer, 1988). Likewise, despite the fact that the first women with immune suppression were noted by the CDC in August 1981 (Oppenheimer, 1988), women with AIDS were usually placed in the more general epidemiological category of "Other," marginalizing the impact of AIDS on their lives (Treichler, 1988). Finally, a last reason for the strong AIDS/gay link in the news may have been that the nature of news—the tendency to collapse information and to make the complex simple (especially in headlines)—would seem to exclude exceptions about the gay nature of AIDS. Scientific research is complex, and this complexity must be made simple in news. One way to do this is to leave out some of the complexity, such as the finding of exceptions or anomalies in research. With AIDS, such tendencies strengthened the "pure" relationship between gays and AIDS. Albert (1986b) argued that one effect of this linkage is to imply that biological differences between gays and straights (i.e., gays are unhealthy) exist where only behavioral differences existed before.

But even if the link between AIDS and gays was impossible to break, news coverage of AIDS could still be beneficial to gays if this coverage was sympathetic to those afflicted. However, early news reports of AIDS tended to stress the "deviant" nature of people who suffered from immune suppression. Therefore, not only was there a strong link created between a disease and a demographic group in the news (AIDS and gay men), but also cultural meanings and cultural judgments were imposed upon that link. In the news, AIDS became a metaphor for gay men and for those who violated social norms.

The journalist's goal of making the strange familiar was discussed earlier. With some items, however, this is perceived as impossible: The only way to make the strange understandable to readers is to emphasize its strangeness even more. It appears that this technique was most chosen for AIDS narratives. News stories emphasized that gays with AIDS were indeed strange (in fact, the reason they had AIDS was because they were strange), and so readers should understand them as strange. Stressing the "unusual" became the newsworthy slant of AIDS.

Thus, many early portrayals stressed the "non-normative" sex practices of those gay men afflicted with immune suppression (Albert, 1986b). In this case, "promiscuity" became the defining property. This image of gay men with AIDS, in fact, fit into the already established stereotypes of gay lifestyle (Seidman, 1988). Stories examined in depth (although constrained by the language of good taste) the stereotypical gay lifestyle, for example its emphasis on "fast lane sex" and recreational drugs. As Albert (1986b) noted, equivalent examinations of the effect of lifestyle were not given to those afflicted by Legionnaire's Disease or by toxic-shock syndrome. With people with AIDS it was their "strange" nature that made the lifestyle factors relevant and newsworthy. Perhaps the most notorious example of a news item that highlighted the alien nature of gays was Patrick Buchanan's editorial in the New York *Post,* entitled "AIDS Disease: It's Nature Striking Back" (cited in Altman, 1986).

Why were the "deviant" aspects of gay life emphasized to such a large degree, and what effect did this emphasis have? Part of the reason that the stereotypes of gay lifestyle were so stressed was that the medical sources used by news stressed these elements as well. Thus, one early medical hypothesis linking stereotypical gay lifestyles to disease focused on the use of stimulants like amyl nitrite, or "poppers," by some gay men to increase their sexual pleasure (Oppenheimer, 1988). Another theory concentrated on the perceived promiscuousness of gay males, advocating that some overly sexual bodies reached an "overload" stage, making them especially susceptible to disease (Altman, 1986). Also, however, stressing such elements helped to sell papers. As Altman (1986) argued, "Medical stories are particularly attractive to the media, and where they can be linked to both high fatalities and stigmatized sexuality we have all the ingredients for banner headlines" (p. 19).

Such a linkage of AIDS with negative images of gays may have several consequences. The strength of the deviant gay/AIDS association perhaps affected how people viewed AIDS. For example, one effect of the stress on gays' deviant image was to cause a "slippage" in meaning in which the categories gay and promiscuous and AIDS are collapsed together (Watney, 1987). Also, such coverage may lead to a lack of identification with people with AIDS. Obviously, stressing the deviance of those afflicted would discourage identification (i.e., "Gays are not like us").

Critiques of news coverage, however, have pointed to other elements in news coverage that rhetorically undermine reader identification with those with AIDS. For example, scholars have noted the creation of a "victim continuum" for people with AIDS, which distinguishes the "innocent victims" from the "guilty victims" (Albert, 1986a, 1986b; Karpf, 1988; Patton, 1985; Treichler, 1987, 1988; Watney, 1986, 1987). On one end of the continuum are those "innocent" people, those portrayed as guiltless bystanders who, through no fault of their own (in fact, maybe even through the fault of others), have contracted AIDS. On the opposite end are guilty victims, those whose conscious behavior has led to the disease. Albert (1986a) discussed how news places children at the innocent end, Haitians in the middle, and gays and drug users at the guilty end. Photos accompanying the news stories tend to reinforce this continuum. Children with AIDS are pictured with people who do not wear protective gear, whereas other people with AIDS are not (Albert, 1986b). Treichler (1988), likewise, described how certain "innocent" people with AIDS—or physicians working on AIDS—tend to be "normalized" in photographs: Children with AIDS are pictured with stuffed or live animals, and physicians working on AIDS are pictured with their families.

Another narrative technique that discourages identification with people with AIDS was the early emphasis on "panic in the streets" (Albert, 1986a, 1986b). The gay community was portrayed in the news media as enveloped by a "reign of terror." For most readers of mass circulation newspapers, however, the everyday effects of AIDS could not be seen, especially in the early years. By stressing the "panic," Albert (1986a) concluded, the AIDS phenomenon was framed as distant, "like a famine in Africa or an earthquake far away" (p. 148).

Finally, Watney (1986) observed that gay individuals with AIDS were placed in specific "roles" in early news, roles that complemented the stereotype of the promiscuous gay lifestyle. The first "role" is that of the gay man who has been abandoned to die by his gay lover and friends. Second, there is the image of the gay man with AIDS who continues to have casual "unsafe" sex despite his knowledge of infection. Finally, the third role Watney delineated, the most frequent and pathetic role, is one in which a frail, dying AIDS patient denounces his former lifestyle. An example of this third role may be found in a 1982 issue of *Us* magazine, which relates the story of a gay man with AIDS who tells his nurse that "if I pull through I promise I'll find a girlfriend" (quoted in Altman, 1986).

As Watney concluded, "A disease of chimpanzees or gerbils would have attracted more sympathetic coverage" (p. 47).

Related to the "AIDS-as-metaphor" medicalized tendency, a second characteristic of AIDS coverage that illustrates the influence of medicalized perspectives has been a dependence on medical sources in AIDS stories.

AIDS Coverage and Medical Dependence

Certain medical organizations and medical journals basically controlled the amount of information in the news about AIDS, and the type of information. The CDC, for example, was the main source of information during the first year or so for many newspapers: Often AIDS would not have been mentioned at all if not for CDC press releases (Schwartz, 1984). In fact, it could be argued that one reason that AIDS was not mentioned for long periods of time in these early years was because the CDC's publication, the *Morbidity and Mortality Weekly Report* (MMWR), did not publish any new updates for months at a time (Kinsella, 1989). Also, as discussed earlier, because the CDC in these early years tended to stress epidemiology, news stories emphasized the "who" element over other news elements (Albert, 1986a).

But perhaps with even more ability to generate publicity and place news stories about AIDS were the "prestige" hard science journals like the *New England Journal of Medicine* (NEJM) and the *Journal of the American Medical Association* (JAMA). Kinsella (1989) pointed out that the very first discussion about AIDS on national television (lasting 45 seconds) took place on ABC's "Good Morning America" after the December 10, 1981 issue of NEJM addressed the topic. Thus, despite the fact that New York, Los Angeles, and San Francisco were the three main cities affected by AIDS, the reliance on the main medical research outlets such as journals and conferences meant that stories from the wire services like Associated Press (AP) often originated from Atlanta (the location of the CDC), from Washington, DC, and even from Daytona Beach where the topic was discussed at an American Cancer Society conference (Kinsella, 1989). One reporter for AP relied so heavily on such medical research sources that he still had not met a person with AIDS after a year and a half covering the topic (Kinsella, 1989).

In a similar manner, the "casual contact" hypothesis appearing in the May 6, 1983 issue of JAMA sparked increased coverage of AIDS. In this issue of JAMA, an editorial by Anthony S. Fauci of the National Institutes of Health fueled fear by speculating on the likelihood of transmitting AIDS through "routine casual contact" (Fauci, 1983). Although this hypothesis was later discredited, the fact that this hypothesis appeared in an established medical journal is crucial in understanding how news uses medical and scientific sources. As Schwartz (1984) observed,

> Once a seemingly authoritative source such as the *Journal* raised the specter that AIDS was not necessarily limited to a few specific groups, many in the media felt they had important backing to speculate and to scare. (p. 93)

In fact, by looking at *The New York Times Index,* one finds that from July 1981 to March 1983 there were 18 articles about AIDS published in *The New York Times*; in the next 3 months, the period during which the JAMA issue mentioned earlier was published, 49 articles about AIDS appeared in the newspaper.

As medical science began to discuss the nature of AIDS with more confidence—as "hard science" took over from the epidemiologists—its power as a source for AIDS issues was granted longevity. Albert (1986a) suggested that between May 1982 and December 1984 there was a very definite shift from stories that stressed "lifestyle" to those that stressed "science." Stories, then, went from in-depth descriptions of "gay lifestyle" (although the association was already very strong) to stories about "the medical detective," climaxing in the discovery of the virus and viral tests. Such a shift further implied that science was getting to the heart of the matter, which served to "rationalize the threat, i.e. normalize it, for the population at large" (Albert, 1986a, p. 153).

Also, medicine proved to be a useful source in that it provided a printable vocabulary. Although AIDS might help sell newspapers because of its sexual nature, it could also bring criticism because of the words used to describe its sexual nature. Biomedicine helps to solve this problem somewhat. Medical language is safe, while certain expressions coming from the gay community (like "fisting") were considered, especially early in the phenomenon, too risky for publication (Leff & Adolph, 1986). In fact, it was only when medical sources began using more explicit language that reporters felt comfortable with including this language in their stories (Leff & Adolph, 1986). One illustration of this occurred in 1985, when ABC reporter George Strait asked Dr. Anthony Fauci of the National Institute of Health "to use the term 'anal sex' on the air so the reporter would not have to" (Kinsella, 1989, p. 136).

AIDS seems to be fertile ground for increased celebration and use of medical professional and ideological authority in the news. But are there counter-elements in the relationship between AIDS and medicine that may encourage criticisms of medicine to be placed in the news? May AIDS actually contain factors that encourage demedicalization? The following subsection addresses this question.

AIDS, News, and the Possibilities
for Demedicalization

Despite the factors just discussed, AIDS also has the potential to lead to a
questioning of the role of medicine—a "demedicalization"—at both the
biomedical research level and the health-care delivery level, and this question does occasionally find its place in the news media. At the level of research, as Altman (1986) pointed out, AIDS has created a scrutiny and
accountability of medical research that is unprecedented. The highly publicized nature of AIDS, the desire of many groups to meet with medical
researchers, and the willingness of such researchers to "publicize" their
names has created public forums, conferences, and meetings. Berk (1987)
hypothesized that such high visibility could lead to high expectations,
with the result being that if no cure is found, science will be blamed for
wastefully spending millions of dollars. Also, such visibility could reveal
insights into the biomedical research process, a revealing that could go
far in "demystifying" medical research. A high degree of accessibility to
the medical research system could help reveal "hidden agendas" in the
system, agendas influenced by moral or economic imperatives. So, for
example, the conflict between Drs. Robert C. Gallo of the National Cancer
Institute and Luc Montagnier of the Institute Pasteur in France over who
discovered the virus associated with AIDS revealed the politics and economics of biomedical scientific research. It may be the most publicized
scientific dispute in the last 20 years. The *Chicago Tribune* devoted an
entire section of its Sunday paper (November 19, 1989), entailing 50,000
words and 16 pages, to "The Great AIDS Quest" (Crewsdon, 1989).

Health-care delivery may also experience a certain degree of vulnera-
bility because of AIDS. Certain shortcomings in the American medical system (preferences for the rich, tendencies to "dump" problem patients,
discrimination in health care) could be revealed with the increased use
of health-care facilities that AIDS brings (Altman, 1986). With the increasing number of people with AIDS, and the strain on the medical system
these numbers cause, the before-concealed "cracks" in the medical system could open up to become crevasses.

Finally, the gay and lesbian community—a community traditionally
very critical of medicine—could become more unified and powerful as
it deals with AIDS issues. As the power of the community increases, so
may its ability to provide alternatives to mainstream health care, and so
may its voice criticizing medicine and other institutions it views as op-
pressive. Patton (1985) noted that:

> Lesbian/gay health care will never be the same: the increase in awareness
> of sex-related health issues and the sense of empowerment about commu-

nity control of sexuality and health, despite the tragic destruction of AIDS, will move sexually related health care problems to a more acknowledged status. (p. 144)

Of course, the most publicized example of such criticism of medicine may be found in the activities of the group AIDS Coalition to Unleash Power (ACT-UP), a group whose membership includes gays and straights. ACT-UP and groups like it are very sophisticated in their ability to generate publicity and to place news stories criticizing dominant decision-making powers involved with AIDS, including medicine. By using "guerilla theater" tactics, and producing their own posters and advertisements, such groups offer a vehicle for continual public criticism of medicine (see Crimp with Rolston, 1990; Treichler, 1991; for discussions and examples of such criticism).

This chapter has attempted to describe the applicability of one critical approach toward medicine, medicalization, to understanding the nature of news coverage of AIDS. It was hypothesized that given some structural qualities of mainstream news, stories about AIDS would be especially susceptible to medicalized coverage. However, although medical authority is powerful in stories about AIDS, its power is not absolute, and oftentimes "leaks" in this power may encourage medical criticism.

What the perspective of medicalization may offer to communication scholars is a critical framework with which to understand some of the implications of communication and health. Is it the sole goal of communication researchers, for example, to increase the communicative efficiency of physicians and health professionals? Or should communication scholars view issues of health in the same light as issues of race, gender, and class? Medicalization reminds those who work in health communication that social power is a pervasive part of life, even in such a seemingly "neutral" area of making people well.

Future research in mass-mediated health communication, then, could strive to refine the usefulness of medicalization in understanding news coverage. Are there specific times when coverage is less medicalized than others, and why? Are there specific subtopics of AIDS (e.g., the development of an AIDS vaccine, or children and AIDS) that are more likely to be medicalized than others? Are there specific types of news (print vs. broadcast; general vs. specialized) that lend themselves to more medicalized types of authority than others? Finally, what is the effect of medicalized and nonmedicalized news coverage of AIDS? Answering such questions may help us to understand better the relationship between the news institution and the medical institution, and the nature of medical news coverage.

ACKNOWLEDGMENTS

This chapter is derived from my doctoral dissertation, "Medicalization in the news media: A comparison of AIDS coverage in three newspapers" (University of Illinois at Urbana-Champaign, 1990). The chapter was presented at the 41st annual meeting of the International Communication Association, Chicago, Illinois, May 1991. I wish to thank D. Charles Whitney, Clifford G. Christians, John C. Nerone, and Paula A. Treichler for their helpful comments on earlier versions of this chapter.

REFERENCES

Albert, E. (1986a). Acquired Immune Deficiency Syndrome: The victim and the press. *Studies in Communication, 3,* 135–158.

Albert, E. (1986b). Illness and deviance: The response of the press to AIDS. In D. A. Feldman & T. M. Johnson (Eds.), *The social dimensions of AIDS: Method and theory* (pp. 163–178). New York: Praeger.

Altman, D. (1986). *AIDS in the mind of America.* Garden City, NY: Anchor Press.

Baker, A. J. (1986). The portrayal of AIDS in the media: An analysis of articles in the *New York Times.* In D. A. Feldman & T. M. Johnson (Eds.), *The social dimensions of AIDS: Method and theory* (pp. 179–194). New York: Praeger.

Barker-Benfield, G. J. (1978). Sexual surgery in late-nineteenth century America. In C. Dreifus (Ed.), *Seizing our bodies: The politics of women's health* (pp. 13–41). New York: Vintage Books.

Bayer, R. (1981). *Homosexuality and American psychiatry: The politics of diagnosis.* New York: Basic Books.

Bennett, W. L. (1988). *News: The politics of illusion.* New York: Longman.

Berk, R. A. (1987). Anticipating the social consequences of AIDS: A position paper. *The American Sociologist, 18*(3), 211–227.

Brandt, A. M. (1988). AIDS: From social history to social policy. In E. Fee & D. M. Fox (Eds.), *AIDS: The burdens of history* (pp. 147–171). Berkeley: University of California Press.

Calnan, M. (1984). Women and medicalisation: An empirical examination of the extent of women's dependence on medical technology in the early detection of breast cancer. *Social Science and Medicine, 18,* 561–569.

Carey, J. W. (1987). The dark continent of American journalism. In R. K. Manoff & M. Schudson (Eds.), *Reading the news* (pp. 146–196). New York: Pantheon.

Clarke, J. N. (1984). Medicalization and secularization in selected English Canadian fiction. *Social Science and Medicine, 18*(3), 205–210.

Conrad, P. (1980). Implications of changing social policy for the medicalization of deviance. *Contemporary Crises, 4*(2), 195–205.

Conrad, P., & Schneider, J. W. (1980). *Deviance and medicalization: From badness to sickness.* St. Louis: C. V. Mosby.

Crawford, R. (1980). Healthism and the medicalization of everyday life. *International Journal of Health Services, 10*(3), 365–388.

Crewsdon, J. (1989, November 19). The great AIDS quest. *Chicago Tribune,* pp. E1–E16.

Crimp, D., with Rolston, A. (1990). *AIDS demographics.* Seattle: Bay Press.

Cronholm, M., & Sandell, R. (1981). Scientific information: A review of research. *Journal of Communication, 31*(2), 85–96.

Dornan, C. (1990). Some problems in conceptualizing the issue of "science and the media." *Critical Studies in Mass Communication, 7*(1), 48–71.

Dunwoody, S. (1980). The science writing inner club: A communication link between science and the lay public. *Science, Technology, & Human Values, 5*(30), 14–22.

Dunwoody, S., & Ryan, M. (1987). The credible scientific source. *Journalism Quarterly, 64,* 21–27.

Ehrenreich, B., & English, D. (1978). Complaints and disorders: The sexual politics of sickness. In C. Dreifus (Ed.), *Seizing our bodies: The politics of women's health* (pp. 43–56). New York: Vintage Books.

Engelhardt, H. T., Jr. (1986). *The foundations of bioethics.* New York: Oxford University Press.

Fauci, A. S. (1983). The Acquired Immune Deficiency Syndrome: The ever-broadening clinical spectrum. *Journal of the American Medical Association, 249,* 2375–2376.

Fisher, J., Gandy, O. H., & Janus, N. Z. (1981). The role of popular media in defining sickness and health. In E. G. McAnany, J. Schnitman, & N. Z. Janus (Eds.), *Communication and social structure* (pp. 240–257). New York: Praeger.

Folland, S. T. (1985). The effects of health care advertising. *Journal of Health Politics, Policy and Law, 10*(2), 329–345.

Foucault, M. (1975). *The birth of the clinic: An archeology of medical perception.* New York: Vintage Books.

Foucault, M. (1977). *Madness and civilization: A history of insanity in the age of reason.* London: Tavistock.

Fox, D. M. (1988). AIDS and the American health polity: The history and prospects of a crisis of authority. In E. Fee & D. M. Fox (Eds.), *AIDS: The burdens of history* (pp. 316–343). Berkeley: University of California Press.

Fox, R. C. (1977). The medicalization and demedicalization of American society. *Daedalus, 106*(1), 9–22.

Gandy, O. H. (1982). *Beyond agenda setting: Information subsidies and public policy.* Norwood, NJ: Ablex.

Gans, H. J. (1979). *Deciding what's news: A study of CBS Evening News, NBC Nightly News, Newsweek, and Time.* New York: Pantheon Books.

Getz, J. G., & Hawkins, R. (1979, Spring). Medicalization as carcinogen. *Sociological Forum,* 4–20.

Goffman, E. (1961). *Asylums: Essays on the social situation of mental patients and other inmates.* Garden City, NY: Anchor Books.

Hall, S., Critcher, C., Jefferson, T., Clarke, J., & Roberts, B. (1978). *Policing the crisis: Mugging, the state, and law and order.* New York: Holmes & Meier.

Hughey, J. D., Norton, R. W., & Sullivan, C. (1986, November). *Confronting danger: AIDS in the news.* Paper presented at the meeting of the Speech Communication Association, Chicago, IL.

Illich, I. (1976). *Medical nemesis: The expropriation of health.* New York: Bantam Books.

Karpf, A. (1988). *Doctoring the media: The reporting of health and medicine.* New York: Routledge, Chapman & Hall.

Katz, J., & Abel, C. F. (1984). The medicalization of repression: Eugenics and crime. *Contemporary Crises, 8*(3), 227–241.

Kinsella, J. (1989). *Covering the plague: AIDS and the American media.* New Brunswick, NJ: Rutgers University Press.

Knowles, J. H. (1977). Introduction. *Daedalus, 106*(1), 1–7.

Leff, L., & Adolph, J. (1986, March/April). AIDS and the family paper. *Columbia Journalism Review,* pp. 11–12.

Mark, V. H., Sweet, W. H., & Ervin, F. R. (1967). Role of brain disease in riots and urban violence. *Journal of the American Medical Association, 201*(11), 217.

Molotch, H., & Lester, M. (1974). Accidents, scandals, and routines: Resources for insurgent methodology. In G. Tuchman (Ed.), *The TV establishment: Programming for power and profit* (pp. 53–65). Englewood Cliffs, NJ: Prentice-Hall.

Navarro, V. (1975). The industrialization of fetishism or the fetishism of industrialization: A critique of Ivan Illich. *Social Science and Medicine, 9,* 351–363.

Nelkin, D. (1985). Managing biomedical news. *Social Research, 52*(3), 625–646.

Nelkin, D. (1987). *Selling science: How the press covers science and technology.* New York: W. H. Freeman.

Oppenheimer, G. M. (1988). In the eye of the storm: The epidemiological construction of AIDS. In E. Fee & D. M. Fox (Eds.), *AIDS: The burdens of history* (pp. 267–300). Berkeley: University of California Press.

Parsons, T. (1951). *The social system.* New York: The Free Press.

Patton, C. (1985). *Sex and germs: The politics of AIDS.* Boston: South End Press.

Pence, G. (1989). Evaluative assumptions and facts about AIDS. In J. M. Humber & R. F. Almeder (Eds.), *Biomedical ethics reviews* (pp. 5–19). Clifton, NJ: Humana Press.

Pfund, N., & Hofstadter, L. (1981). Biomedical innovation and the press. *Journal of Communication, 31*(2), 138–154.

Pitts, J. (1968). Social control: The concept. In D. Sills (Ed.), *International encyclopedia of the social sciences* (Vol. 14, pp. 381–396). New York: Macmillan.

Riessman, C. K. (1983). Women and medicalization: A new perspective. *Social Policy, 14*(1), 3–18.

Robbins, T., & Anthony, D. (1982). Deprogramming, brainwashing, and the medicalization of deviant religious groups. *Social Problems, 29*(3) 283–297.

Roman, P. (1980). Medicalization and social control in the workplace: Prospect of the 1980s. *The Journal of Applied Behavioral Science, 16*(3), 407–422.

Ruzek, S. B. (1978). *The women's health movement: Feminist alternatives to medical control.* New York: Praeger.

Schwartz, H. (1984). AIDS in the media. In *Science in the streets: A report to the Twentieth Century Task Force on the Communication of Scientific Risk* (pp. 87–97). New York: Priority Press.

Seidman, S. (1988). Transfiguring sexual identity: AIDS and the contemporary construction of homosexuality. *Social Text, 19/20,* 187–205.

Shoemaker, P. J. (1987). The communication of deviance. In B. Dervin & M. J. Voigt (Eds.), *Progress in the communication sciences* (Vol. 8, pp. 151–175). Norwood, NJ: Ablex.

Sigal, L. V. (1973). *Reporters and officials: The organization and politics of newsmaking.* Lexington, MA: Heath.

Silverman, D. (1988). *Communication and medical practice: Social relations in the clinic.* Beverly Hills: Sage.

Sontag, S. (1979). *Illness as metaphor.* New York: Vintage Books.

Sontag, S. (1988). *AIDS and its metaphors.* New York: Farrar, Straus, & Giroux.

Stewart, M., & Roter, D. (1989). *Communicating with medical patients.* Beverly Hills: Sage.

Szasz, T. S. (1961). *The myth of mental illness: Foundations of a theory of personal conduct.* New York: Hoeber-Harper.

Szasz, T. S. (1970). *The manufacture of madness: A comparative study of the Inquisition and the mental health movement.* New York: Dell.

Treichler, P. A. (1987). AIDS, homophobia, and biomedical discourse: An epidemic of signification. *Cultural Studies, 1*(3), 263–305.

Treichler, P. A. (1988). AIDS, gender, and biomedical discourse: Current contests for meaning. In E. Fee & D. M. Fox (Eds.), *AIDS: The burdens of history* (pp. 190–266). Berkeley: University of California Press.

Treichler, P. A. (1990). Feminism, medicine, and the meaning of childbirth. In M. Jacobus, E. F. Keller, & S. Shuttleworth (Eds.), *Body/politics: Women and the discourses of science* (pp. 113–138). New York: Routledge.

Treichler, P. A. (1991). How to have theory in an epidemic: The evolution of AIDS treatment activism. In C. Penley & A. Ross (Eds.), *Technoculture.* Minneapolis: University of Minnesota Press.

Tuchman, G. (1978). *Making news: A study in the construction of reality.* New York: The Free Press.

Watney, S. (1986). Common knowledge. *High Performance, 36*(4), 44–47.

Watney, S. (1987). *Policing desire: Pornography, AIDS, and the media.* Minneapolis: University of Minnesota Press.

Winsten, J. A. (1985). Science and the media: The boundaries of truth. *Health Affairs, 4*(1), 5–23.

Zola, I. K. (1972). Medicine as an institution of social control. *Sociological Review, 20,* 487–504.

Author Index

Subject Index